NATURAL HAIR FOR YOUNG WOMEN

A STEP-BY-STEP GUIDE TO NATURAL HAIR FOR BLACK WOMEN, THE BEST HAIR PRODUCTS, HAIR GROWTH, HAIR TREATMENTS, NATURAL HAIR STYLIST, NATURAL HAIR SALONS, NATURAL HAIR STYLES, COLORING NATURAL HAIR, AND ALL THINGS PERTAINING TO BLACK NATURAL HAIR

PHYLECIA TARAEL-ANU

ANU PUBLISHING

ISBN-13: 978-0615825885 (ANU Publishing)

Natural Hair for Young Women
Phylecia Tarael-ANU
iHairNatural
iHiarNatural.com
ISBN-13: 978-0615825885 (ANU PUBLISHING)
ISBN-10: 0615825885

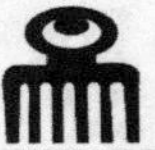 

Dedication:

I dedicate this work to my Ori, Egun, and the Orisas. Thank you for your guidance and support in helping me to bring this work from the unseen to the seen.

To my family; for being the conduit from which I came. I am thankful for the lessons that I continue to learn from and through you.

To my Dear Divine Light; thank you for being a beautiful spirit and for always being my inspiration. This work would not be possible without you and your grace.

To my future children; for being the driving force behind this creation. This is one of many works to come.

To our young women who are shifting towards a more natural way of being; I will that this work will provide a spark of light along your journey.

To the iHairNatural.com community; thank you for being supportive of this work and for sharing your personal gems with myself and our blossoming young women.

To Nature; I am finally listening!

CONTENTS

CHAPTER 1: WHAT IS BLACK NATURAL HAIR?

"The spirit of "doing for self" is now fast coming into our people. They only need a new education of self and other." –Elijah Muhammad

WHAT IS BLACK NATURAL HAIR?

There are plenty of books on the shelves of bookstores that speak to the topic of black natural hair, but has anyone ever taken a moment to explore its actual meaning in order to gain a better understanding of its attributes? Let us take a minute to delve deeper and explore what black natural black hair is. First, let us begin with the word:

BLACK

When one tends to think of the word "black", most people generally think of a color, or the color of a group of people. However, this book is not simply speaking about hair that is black in color, or dyed black, because people of all ethnicities have the potential to produce hair with a black hue. This book is also not referring to people who are considered "black" because of the hue of their skin color, as similarly, people of all different ethnicities would also fall into this category. The people and the type of hair that this book is referring to are not reduced to a simple designation of a color. In order to gain a better understanding and provide some clarity, let us take a look at some meanings of the word "black".

According to the American Heritage College Dictionary, Third Edition. The Latin root of the word black can be defined as follows:

1. *Color, complete or almost complete absence of light; darkness. Being of the color black, producing ...little light...and having no predominate hue. 2. Having little or no light. 3. Often relating to or belonging to a racial group having brown to black skin esp. one of African origin. b. Of, relating to, or belonging to an American ethnic group descended from African peoples having dark skin 4. Very dark in color.*

If we explore the Greek root of the word black, one will find that the word black stems from the root word *melas*, or *melan*, which is where we get the word melanin.

Taking a closer look at the fist definition and how it describes people, one can see that it references descendants of African origin, and the Greek root meaning gives us the word melanin. In terms of the word *"black,"* this book is referring to a people who are melanated and directly from or descendants of the continent of Africa.

However, in contrast to the definition which describes "black" as having *"little or no light"*, the people that this book is referring to are full of light. Light is the source of energy for melanated people. Melanin has an absorbing quality that allows melanated people to consume light and heat energy from the sun, and other rays of light including that of sound. Melanin then stores this light energy within our bodies as fuel which it uses to help sustain, protect, and even heal our bodies. Most of this energy is stored and not projected back out as light, therefore it gives off the reflection of a black color, although the core of this substance consists of pure and divine light. In terms of hair, this book is referring to the natural hair that belongs to this unique group of melanated people. This author also belongs to this group.

Melanin will be further examined in Chapter 2; for now let us take a further look at the word:

NATURAL

According to the **American Heritage College Dictionary**, Third Edition, the Latin root of the word natural can be defined as follows:

Natural: 1. Conforming to the usual or ordinary course of nature. 4a. Not acquired; inherent. 4b. Not produced or changed artificially. 5. Characterized by spontaneity and freedom from artificiality. 6. Not altered, treated or disguised. Faithfully representing nature or life. 13. An Afro hairstyle.

Nature: 3. The world of living things and the outdoors. 4. A primitive state of existence, untouched, and uninfluenced by civilization or artificiality. 7. The essential characteristics or qualities of a person or thing 9. The real aspect of a person place or thing.

From these definitions one can see that something that is natural or related to nature is alive; a living force, therefore hair that is natural is also alive and living. *Natural hair* is not dead as hair is often described in textbooks once it extends beyond the scalp.

Black Natural Hair is Alive

Black natural hair is alive. Its purpose is not simply for warmth or a sun-shield as it is often referenced in textbooks, articles, and informational sites on the internet. It does not lie flat to cover the ears and neck. Black natural hair serves as antennas from which we are able to send and receives messages from the cosmos and between each other. It grows up towards the sun, moon, and the stars, further evidencing our connection to the divine.

Acquired Hair is Not Natural

As referenced in the definition of '*natural*', something that is *acquired or produced artificially* is not natural. This includes hair that is purchased in stores, whether it be synthetic or 100% human hair purchased for wigs or weaving. This type of hair is not living, it is lifeless; dead.

Studies have shown that women have reported that they develop headaches when their hair is not clean. Unclean hair not only contributes to headaches, but it can also restrict the natural flow of one's thoughts and how they send and receive messages. If simply not washing one's hair can have this affect, then wearing something that is dead can limit this exchange as well. It can affect the energy surrounding one's thoughts and the types of messages that are being transmitted. One's thoughts may be dead, lifeless, uncreative, or maybe not even their own.

Hair carries and stores our personal energy. Choosing to wear unnatural forms of hair can cause one to possibly carry someone else's energy. This energy may not be in alignment with their own and may cause internal conflict leading to conflicting thoughts and ideas, confusion and a lack of productivity. This diminishes the capacity of one's spirit and power because it is being used as a conduit by a foreign energy.

Relaxed Hair is Not Natural Hair

According to these definitions one can see that something that is *altered* or *treated*, or *produced* or *changed artificially* is not natural. This includes natural hair that has been chemically relaxed. Having natural hair does not include the process of taking out one's weave to unveil their chemically processed hair. While relaxed hair is a product of hair that grows out of one's scalp, it is not *"Faithfully representing nature or life"* or *"An Afro hairstyle"* as the definition of *natural* implies.

Kemetic Definition of Natural

Kemet is the native name for Ancient Egypt. Kemet translates into the word "Land of the Burnt Faces." According to the Kemetic definition, the word nature is derived from the word NTR or Neter. One can see the word "nurture" has its roots from the word NTR as well.

This definition refers to all living natural things such as birds, flowers, the sky etc. This definition also reveres things that are considered natural as divine or god-like, therefore when one is in alignment with nature and with what is natural, they are holistically and spiritually in alignment with the divine. Our mind, body, and spirit are all connected; harm to one harms the others. For this reason, one's entire being should be honored and nurtured; down to the strands of their hair.

HAIR

Natural hair is what is referred to as a *"crown."* This is not simply because it lies on top of one's head, but because for melanated people the crown signifies royalty and ruler-ship. Ruler-ship, over the planet, and one's entire being.

In Yoruba spiritual systems, the "crown" is one of the locations where the Ori resides. The Ori is the soul; one's highest self. Masking one's crown with unnatural substances, and toxic chemicals is not only hazardous to one's health, but it can diminish one's ability to function to their highest potential. The Ori is our life force; the essence of what we are. Its purpose is to *"assist us in achieving oneness with all of creation while maintaining and strengthening our relationship with our highest order thinking and functioning...our chain link to the supreme intelligence..which allows us to fully realize ourselves as deities."* H. Yuya T. Assaan-ANU, Chief Jegna of the Sadulu House Spiritual Institute, and author of "Grasping the Root of Divine Power."

Wearing natural hair will help one to get back in step with their best self. They will walk in harmony with nature and begin to see their spirit grow, and blossom; exposing the fullness of who and what they are.

CHAPTER 2: MELANIN

His head is as the most fine gold, his locks are bushy, and black as a raven. "The Holy Bible/Song of Solomon 5:11

While we discussed what makes our hair so special and unique, we did not examine one of the key factors that differentiates our hair from any other group of people. This factor also distinguishes the nature of our entire being from *any* other group of individuals on the planet; this key factor is melanin.

Researching definitions of the word melanin, one may find several definitions that are similar to meanings for the word black, where a color or pigment is primarily referenced. If we take a look at the Latin meaning for the word melanin, it is defined as:

Melanin

Any of a group of black or dark brown pigments present in the hair, skin, and eyes of man and animals: produced in excess in certain skin diseases and in melanomas.

Melanin is in Our Hair Skin and Eyes

While this definition is relevant, it is very limited and does not *nearly* cover the scope and depth of what this substance truly is. What is key in this particular definition is that it establishes that melanin is present in the hair, skin, and eyes, however it fails to identify that we are the only people that actually have melanin in our hair, skin, and eyes.

Melanin is derived from the Greek word "melas" or "melanos" which means *black*! The root meaning for the word melanin may be defined as black because it literally is blackness in its purest form. As chlorophyll is the primordial substance that makes plants green, because it literally is the color green, melanin is the primordial substance that makes people black or dark in complexion because melanin is literally the color black.

This explains why our people generally only have hair, eyes or skin in a variation of two colors; black or brown. If we use the color spectrum as a reference, any deviation from the color black shows a deficiency or a lack of melanin in that person or in that particular area of that person's body. For instance, someone who has blue eyes has a lack of melanin in their eyes. A person with blond hair or really light skin has a lack of melanin, or a lower quantity of melanin in those **particular** areas of their bodies. These colors clearly deviate from the color black, and therefore indicate an absence of melanin.

Melanin Properly Defined

Melanin is much more than just a pigment that gives us our complexion or hair color. It is a divine cosmic molecule that can be perfectly described in the words of Dr. Jewell Pookrum, author, and preventive and holistic health physician, as ***"Biological living light....the depths of the universe personified in black people."*** It is important to understand that melanin is not only in our skin, eyes and hair, but that melanin actually runs all throughout our bodies, the planet, and the universe.

In terms of the physical nature within our bodies, melanin is a blue black substance or pigment that derives its power from light and heat energy. This energy is a life force in and of itself. Melanin is reflected in the universe literally as the "black stuff", the darkness, the void, ultimately the source. This dark matter is one of *the* most powerful energies in the universe. This not only establishes the cosmic or divine nature of this substance, but also highlights the connecting link to the divinity of our people. We are celestial beings, literally reflecting the cosmos, and black women emulate that energy and power more than any other force on the planet!

Melanin is Feminine Energy

While we are all an amalgam of feminine and masculine qualities, melanin closely resembles feminine energy. Feminine energy, like melanin, is dark matter, the darkness, the void. It is the energy of the moon. It is magnetic, receptive and yielding. It retracts or goes in, and it is moldable. Melanin absorbs light and heat energy, and light energy is masculine energy, it is the energy of the sun. Masculine energy is electric, it projects outward, and it is expansive.

The relationship between melanin and light is not only symbolic of feminine or masculine qualities, or the natural and complementary relationship between the Black Man and the Black Woman, but it is also symbolic of the womb or feminine energy. It is through this infusion of light into the dark matter that life is created. As perfectly coined by HRU Yuya T. Assaan-ANU, author of *"Grasping the Root of Divine Power"*, ***"Feminine energy is the matter of all creation."***

While both light and dark matter are necessary to join and create life; it is the black woman who is the vessel charged with carrying and shaping that life. Walking in this awareness, and taking this responsibility seriously by honoring one's melanin, will in turn be a reflection of honoring oneself.

Melanin and Relationships

Some women may struggle to reveal their beautiful melanated crowns because they fear that they will not be attractive to the young black men who peak their interest, however a black man who is reflective of his true nature, will always be attracted to his complement; the black woman. This is especially the case if she is also reflecting her true self and her true nature. As we previously discussed, like attracts like.

Once we begin to shed perms, and weaves, embracing the beauty of being natural, one will begin to see flower petals unfold as they blossom into a beautiful black woman. As one begins to elevate one will soon realize that they are no longer attracted to the same type of men that once peaked their interest, particularly the men who do not have the eyes to realize the beauty of a natural crown. Activated melanin plays a role within this change of heart as well.

Melanin is energy that vibrates on frequencies. These vibrations emanate from your body and determine what frequency you are on, depending on either how fast or how slow someone is vibrating. If one is on a higher frequency, he or she will connect with, or be drawn to people or experiences that are also on that higher frequency. Others that are not on the same frequency will simply not be able to see you, as you will be in a sense invisible to them.

Think of some of the changes that you may have already made in your life, and the differences that came as a result of the people that were drawn to you, who may have never noticed that you existed prior to your change. Similarly your experiences will be enhanced as you find yourself no longer interested in unproductive activities that consumed the majority of your time and attention on a daily basis. As you grow and elevate yourself, mentally, physically, and spiritually, your entire being shifts and changes. As you come closer and closer to your true self you realize your natural beauty and power.

Melanin and the Pineal Gland

"Give your brain as much attention as your hair, and you'll be a thousand times better off." - ***Malcolm X***

While one may feel that Malcolm X's sage advice may be a poor selection for a book whose main subject is literally about hair, this quote could not be more seemingly fit, or any further from the truth.

The brain is one of the most vital organs in the body. This organ is the body's control center, where thoughts originate, as well as where our Ori resides. Maintaining the health of this organ is not only critical but essential for the wellness of one's entire being. It is essential to become aware of the consequences that can occur as a result of using chemicals on one's hair.

Just as lotions, and facial products are absorbed into the skin, harsh chemicals that are contained in relaxers, hair dyes, hair glues etc., seep through the skin and get absorbed into the bloodstream. Placing these toxins onto the scalp which sits on top of the brain can have damaging and sometimes irreversible effects on the body. These chemicals can interfere with the functioning and vitality of brain activity, and the production of melanin and the pineal gland.

Melanin is secreted from the pineal gland which resides in the brain. The pineal gland is responsible for regulating how much melanin will be produced within our bodies as well as a host of other functions. According to Dr. Llaila Afrika of *"Nutricide,"*

The pineal gland is also responsible for the behavior of organs, bone growth, energy storage, memory, genetic information, extra sensory perception, as well as hair growth. Dr. Afrika advises:

"Drugs such as cocaine...caffeine...aspirin...can have an effect on melanin and the gland. This includes lye and lye-like chemicals (hair relaxers) skin bleaching agents, and hair depilatory chemicals. Toxins in the pineal gland can result in degenerative diseases such as arthritis, senility, cataracts, cancer, Alzheimer's, diabetes, Parkinson, menopause.. glaucoma, osteoporosis, and arteriosclerosis."

This outlines some of the ways that one can weaken or deteriorate the pineal gland. This also displays how chemicals that are contained in relaxers can damage one's bodily functions just the same as any other drug like cocaine or aspirin, especially with long-term use. Although one drug or chemical may seem less harmful than the other, the damage that results appears to be synonymous.

The pineal gland is also known as the third eye. The third eye is located on the foreheads of our spirit bodies. It is through this eye and our connection to the cosmos that we are able "to see" or have the ability of clairvoyant ESP (Extra Sensory Perception); the ability to see beyond the mundane. For some of us, depending on how activated our melanin is, we can literally see and have access to information that others cannot *without* the use of technology.

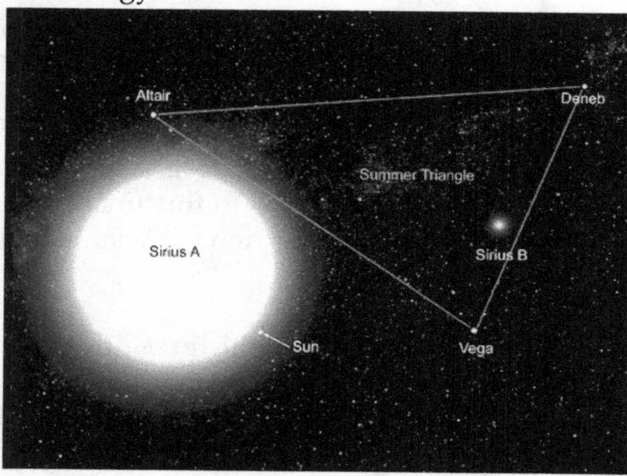

For instance, reports have indicated that the Dogon Tribe of Africa, a highly melanated people, have been able to see constellations of stars with their bare eyes. However, others that

are melanin deficient could only see these constellations with the use of a telescope.
It is through the function of the pineal gland, and melanin, that we are able to connect with our divine nature and abilities. This is also the reason why our people have innate psychic abilities and can also communicate without the use of technology. For instance, we will think of someone, and seconds later they are calling us on the phone. We are telepathic. We have an uncanny ability to know exactly what each other is thinking, especially those who we have a close relationship with. We can talk to each other without the use of words, simply through the use of sounds we have the ability to understand each other. This sensitivity to energy that resides within melanated people is related to the function of melanin and its connection to the cosmos.

According to an interview titled *"The Melanin Chronicles"* featuring Black Studies Professor Dr. Booker T. Coleman, it is through melanin that we have several abilities outside of having extra sensory perception. For instance, it is through melanin that we are able to not only hear voices, but we are able to hear sounds at levels inaudible to the average ear. Accordingly this plays a pivotal role in the musicians ear as he/she is able to pick up the subtle frequencies of sound, and creatively incorporate them into their music.

Dr. Coleman also advises that melanin plays a role in the basketball players ability to jump, as well as the young black woman's ability to jump double dutch, or the singer's ability to sing. There are a myriad of talents that we exhibit that can be attributed to melanin.

Melanin and Healing

Melanin also gives us the ability to heal ourselves. Dr. Jewel Pookrum is a perfect example of this as she was able to heal and cure herself of cancer without the use of drugs or chemotherapy. This is due to the powerful healing abilities of melanin. According to Dr. Coleman our enslaved ancestors who lived on plantations without access to medical attention were able to cure themselves of illness without evening knowing that they were sick. This is because our melanin serves as an agent in the body. Someone who makes an effort to maintain their health and constantly replenish and activate their melanin, will allow the melanin to take on a life of its own. Melanin is able to locate and disintegrate illnesses or diseases such as cancer. The more melanin activity you have, the better the body can automatically protect and heal itself, as well as transmit it where its needed.

How to Activate and Replenish Your Melanin

The Sun

We activate and increase our melanin charge through exposure to the sun. Being highly melanated, and the protective role that melanin plays within our bodies, allows us to be more exposed to the sun than any other group of people. We are protected from the harmful UV rays, and can absorb more sunlight, which in turn gives us the ability to constantly produce more melanin which creates more healing properties inside of our bodies.
Sun exposure is very good for us physically and spiritually. For one, it is one of the most powerful stars in the universe. It is through this warming masculine energy that we are provided with light, as well as with life on our planet. Through constant exposure to the sun we are able to activate the pineal gland. During the day it absorbs energy from the sun and produces serotonin which helps to eliminate waste from the body. At night it produces melatonin and activates our melanin so that we can recharge and regenerate our bodies.

Therefore hairstyles such as perms or weaves that will prevent one from being exposed to the elements such as the sun, due to fear of their perm frizzing out, will not only diminish the quality of one's life, but it will also diminish the quality of one's health and their body's ability to replenish and secrete this powerful substance throughout their body.

In order for one to grow, one must not only learn to exist as they naturally are, but they must also learn to exist in nature. *We have a divine connection with nature, as we are one in the same, and this relationship with nature should be nurtured and integrated within every aspect of our lives.*

The Moon

It is under the moon at night when this amazing substance is activated and aids in the regeneration of our cells. However, this regeneration has to occur in complete darkness with eyes closed shut, therefore make sure that your sleeping environment is entirely absent of light.

How to Nurture Your Melanin

To nurture one's melanin is to nurture yourself by assuring that one is respecting and maintaining the health of their mind, body, and spirit. In terms of diet, melanin effects us differently because of the abundance of melanin within our bodies. Our dietary needs are different from those who are melanin deficient. For this reason we are to use a different standard to measure the quality of our heath. This will be discussed in Chapter 6.

In addition to a healthy diet, one can nurture or increase their melanin by centering themselves around the proper music. This will send vibrations that will balance and heal the energy within one's body. This can also be achieved through meditation, and by repeating mantras such as the popular "om" to aid in re-balancing the energy inside the body. One can also increase their melanin by associating themselves with the proper friends. Proper can be defined by one's spirit, and the frequency that they are on helps as well. If one feels that there is static between their connection and another's, then perhaps it is time to let go of that relationship and join with those on the same frequency or higher in order to maintain a healthy exchange of energy.

It is imperative to understand the important role that the pineal gland and melanin plays within our mental, physical and spiritual being. Melanin is a powerful substance that essentially makes us who we are, therefore it is important to work towards maintaining its vitality versus its deterioration. Chemically relaxed hair is no fare exchange for the gifts and abilities that come along with being a highly functioning melanated being.

CHAPTER 3: 9 ETHER HAIR

"A fruit does not need to be picked from the tree; it is impatience that finds a good taste in a non-ripe fruit." –Nwngu Proverb

"9 Ether Hair" is another concept that reflects our relationship between black natural hair and the universe. However, this concept has its very own unique cosmic expression.

The Powerful Number 9:

In order to gain a basic understanding of what "9 Ether" hair is, let us first examine the number nine. The number nine is the highest number in the mathematical system. It is the last number of the single digits in mathematics (0-9). The number nine illustrates the ending of a series of numbers; however it also denotes the beginning to a next series of numbers. For instance, the following series of numbers would consist of two digits starting with the number one. From this example, one can gather a basic understanding that the number nine indicates a finality, or an ending of a phase, as well as the beginning of a new phase. In other words, the number nine represents an ending or death while simultaneously signifying a beginning or birth.

One can literally examine this point by observing how long it takes to give birth. This is called the gestation period. A full gestation period takes nine months to complete. At this stage a baby is fully formed, at the same time, a new stage has now begun. This new stage for the newborn is to live and function outside of its mother's womb. So again, one can gather how the number nine represents completion, or death and life, as well as a full cycle or circle.

One can explore this concept further by studying the geometric shape of a circle as it relates to the number nine. A circle consists of 360 degrees, and the sum of these numbers is the number nine (3+6+0=9). From this example, one can see how powerful the number nine is. The number nine not only represents man or life, but it also represents a circle (360 degrees) which is a powerful symbol because it identifies completion, as well as life. For example, the atom, the source of life, is in the form of a circle. The cells that roam through our bodies, charged with keeping it fully functioning, healthy and alive are shaped in the form of a circle. The sun that provides life on this planet by providing light, heat, and fire is also shaped in the form of a circle. Most of the prevailing life forms in nature are in the shape of a circle. The mathematical root of these cosmic forces is the number nine.

Through multiplication, we can see how the number nine will constantly reproduce itself. If one were to take the number nine and multiply it by any number, in any variation, the sum of those two numbers would inevitably equate to the number nine. For instance, 9×7=63 and 6+3=9, or 9×5=45 and 4+5=9. Multiply the number nine by every number including itself (9×9=81 and 8+1=9), and it will always come back full circle. Similarly, the same is reflected if a number is added to the number nine. If you take 9+(5)=14 and 4+1=(5) or 9+(2)=11 and 1+1=(2), one can see how adding a number to the number nine does not affect the core common denominator or take away from the number at all. It will always revert to itself as if nothing was added to it. This example portrays the invincible nature of the number nine, which brings us the to the topic of ether.

Ether:

Some Latin root meanings of the word "ether" are defined as:
A colorless, highly volatile, flammable liquid, C 4 H 10 O, having an aromatic odor and sweet, burning taste, derived from ethyl alcohol by the action of sulfuric acid: used as a solvent and, formerly, as an inhalant anesthetic. ....The upper regions of space, the clear sky, the heavens...pure air.

The Greek root meaning of the word ether means to *glow* or to *burn*.

From observing these definitions one can gather that ether is not only a chemical compound or a gas that burns or glows, but it is also the upper regions of space, or the infinite darkness, reflecting the energy of melanin, or the womb from which all things are birthed. Combining this meaning with the number nine, the most powerful life giving number, one can determine that "9 Ether" is the original or the highest life force, as "9 Ether" is the combination of all the existing gases in nature making it the most dynamic. It is said that these powerful combinations of gases create all of existence, life forms, and the planets, solar system, and the sun.

Combining the number 9 and Ether one can see how there is this indestructible life giving force that existed birthing the "beginning", as in life on this planet as well as an end of a phase, which was the completion of the creation of planets in the universe.

What is the Connection with 9 Ether and Our Hair?

Hair that curls is the physical representation of man. The circle or 360 degrees is reflective of the number nine, and life, as it takes nine months to create man. "9 Ether" hair displays how our hair is connected to everything in nature which was created from the "9 Ether" gases. For instance, this explains why our hair is also curly or wooly and grows spiraling up towards the sun and the cosmos, similar to things in nature such as plants, flowers and trees that also grow up towards the sun and the cosmos.

Black natural hair, particularly tightly coiled or "kinky" hair, will literally reflect the shape and supreme energy of the number nine. To determine if you have "9 Ether" hair, simply cut off a small strand of your natural hair, and stretch it out slowly; you will see the number nine constantly repeated throughout the strand. Even if you are natural and wear your hair in the very short almost bald style, you will see the number nine reflected there as well. Simply hold a mirror to the top of your head, and you will see the 9 spiraling throughout the top of your crown. It is almost reflective of a galaxy, or a planet of its own. Even if you have a particularly short cropped natural, or an extremely short afro, the smallest curl will reflect the 360 degrees.

While there are different levels of ether hair, this book will not cover the other levels in detail[1]. A basic understanding is that 9 Ether is the highest, and this is specifically embodied in the natural kinks and curls that most of us have when our hair is in its natural state. "6 Ether" hair is the lowest form. Without even exploring the minute details of "6

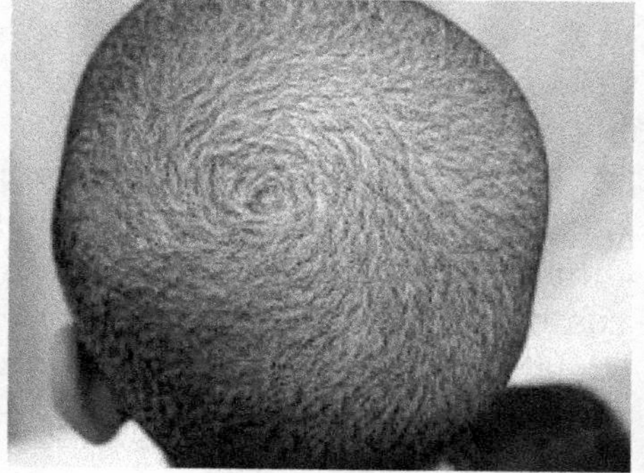

Ether" hair, we can infer from simply observing the shape of the number 6 that it is the complete opposite of "9 Ether" hair, as the number 6 is literally the number 9 upside down. Presumably, this hair type would be the opposite in terms of its nature, structure and energy to "9 Ether" hair.

If someone has altered the natural state of their hair with chemicals like perms, their hair will reflect the characteristics of "6 Ether"; hair that is straight like permed hair. This hair is void of the driving life force that is connected to "9 Ether" hair. It is essentially absent of life; spiritless. One would strip their hair of its natural essence and power.

However, "9 Ether" hair is so powerful in melanated people that it does assert itself to a degree even in permed hair. When one's perm reaches the stage of new growth, one can see how true hair will revert to its natural state, month after month, similar to how the number nine in mathematics will come back full circle to reproduce itself again and again. It usually takes about nine months to grow a perm completely out of the hair, again representing an ending of a phase and the beginning of one returning back to their natural self. *This is another example of how powerful black natural hair is and how deeply connected we are to the divine cosmic forces that exist within our entire being; down to the structure of our hair.*

---

[1]***The levels of Ether Hair are: 9 Ether=Kinky, 8 Ether=Curly, 7 Ether=Wavy and 6 Ether=Straight. For more information about Ether hair please visit www.ihairnatural.com/***

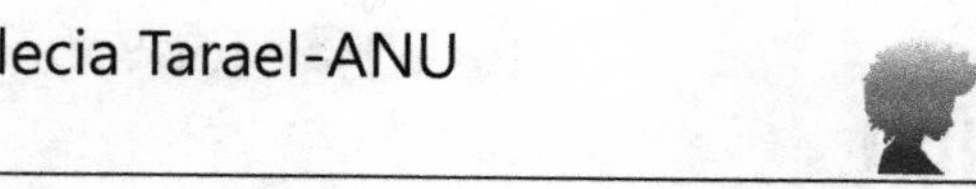

CHAPTER 4: THE HISTORY OF OUR HAIR

"I come from nothing. I depend on nothing. I am the intense flame that is before all things created. I am the will to be."
-Interpretation of Nanan-Bouclou by H. Yuya T. Assaan-ANU

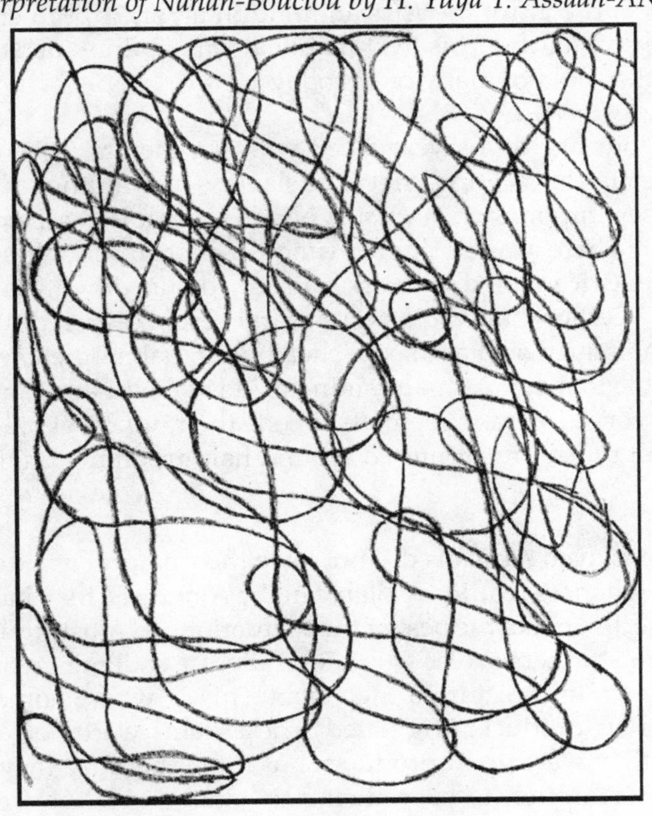

Now that we have covered some of the basic qualities of black natural hair, as well as some of the spiritual aspects; let us explore the history of our hair.

Slavery and Our Hair

When our ancestors fell victim to european enslavement, one of the first things that was done to African royalty; kings, queens, princesses, warriors, and Africans in general, was that they were stripped of their adornments, and many of them had their heads shaved. Our ancestor's natural hair and adornments gave them a tremendous sense of pride, and also served as a form of communication and tribal identification. For instance, hair worn loose indicated that one was mourning, while locs or braided patterns could identify one's tribe, their role within the tribe, as well as their marital status. Removal of these symbols of pride and power was a tactic used in slavery to psychologically breakdown, and control the African mind in an attempt to create the "slave mentality". This dysfunctional way of thinking still exists and takes hold of many of us today.

When our ancestors were faced with the mental, spiritual, and physically devastating effects of slavery, hair aesthetics became of lesser importance, and surviving or escaping became paramount. There was not much time for hair grooming since enslaved Africans had to work sun up to sun down, on a daily basis. Certain hair tools and natural resources used to groom their hair such as black soap, shea butter, palm oil etc. were not available to them. As maintaining pride in their hair waned, they wore scarves or handkerchiefs to hide their unkempt hair. There was not much time centered around hair grooming on the plantations.

Since enslaved Africans did not have their natural resources and hair appliances readily available in the Americas, they had to improvise and make the best of their situation. To substitute for natural moisturizers slaves would literally use cooking grease, lard, butter etc. to moisturize their hair. This is where some myths about hair products originated. These items were not used because they were good products, but rather because they were a last resort option to keep their hair manageable. However, interestingly enough, some 400 hundred years later, some women still put grease in their hair, although we are no longer on slave plantations, and have access to healthier and natural options.

As efforts to abolish slavery commenced, this gave our ancestors a false sense, or an illusion of freedom and new opportunity. Many equated conforming to the local standards of european aesthetics with upward mobility. Light skin, and straight hair, were associated with beauty, freedom, and opportunity. This was beat into the psyche of the enslaved African, while curly, kinky hair, and dark skin were associated with inferiority, and maltreatment by white europeans. During this time, pride in our natural hair and locs ended, and the introduction of toxic chemicals were used in an attempt to look like and mimic the european's straight hair texture. Even more surprisingly, when slavery ended Black Americans increasingly used chemicals to straighten their hair, perfecting old methods. Madame C. J. Walker introduced the very toxic and dangerous chemical we refer to as a perm or relaxer. During this time, wearing the hair in its natural state was outlawed in some cities like New Orleans, where women who chose to wear their hair natural had to wear scarves to cover it. Wearing natural hairstyles declined significantly as Blacks tried to assimilate and conform to the standards of european beauty in an effort to seek out opportunities for advancement. This mental programming was so full proof that some 400 years later many Black women still wear perms and relaxers, and oddly enough some do for the very same reasons.

The Slave Mentality

The slave mentality is one where an individual may be physically free of bondage, but mentally subservient to the domination of some influence, or person. In most cases, one who has the slave mentality is under the influence of those in control of this society. This mentality is often exhibited in descendants of enslaved Africans because of long term dependence on the ruling class that occurred after generations of slavery. While chattel slavery does not exist today, one may still be scared to exist and think freely out of fear of rejection, punishment, or a low sense of self-worth. They may also reject themselves in order to conform and assimilate into mainstream society, as a means of survival.

The media is one of the tools used to replace chattel slavery and perpetuate this slave mentality. It is a powerful tool that is used to program and control the subconscious mind. Commercials, movies, and TV shows dictate to the masses how they should think; what they should eat; what they should buy; what is beautiful; unattractive; essentially how one should think and live their life. This way of being is typically not questioned and becomes conditioned behavior.

This conditioned behavior contributes to why one may come from a generation of women who have permed hair. In many cases it is more than just an issue of manageability, or style preference. It is often behavior that goes unquestioned for years, even decades. Subconsciously it becomes a form of assimilation or a means of survival, out of fear of rejection, or a lack of self-acceptance. This is quite understandable when one lives in a society where they are bombarded by images of "beauty" that don't reflect their own. However, the good news is that it is never too late to break free. Freedom is simply a choice that can be obtained with just a shift of consciousness. Where the mind goes, the body follows. This course of action will begin to break the conditioning and mental programming so that one can take the necessary steps towards freedom; freedom to rule their own mind, and to exist as they naturally are, and create their own standards of beauty.

Cornrows and Braids

Prior to slavery, our ancestors embraced and were proud of their natural curls and kinks which were also worn by kings, queens, warriors; African royalty. Today, several cultures wear braids or cornrows, and without question this practice originated in Africa. These styles can be seen worn by both men and women across the entire African continent, as well as across the globe. Today it appears that many of the techniques originated from West Africa, but evidence of hair braiding dates back to our ancient ancestors. There are images of African sculptures which date back to 2000

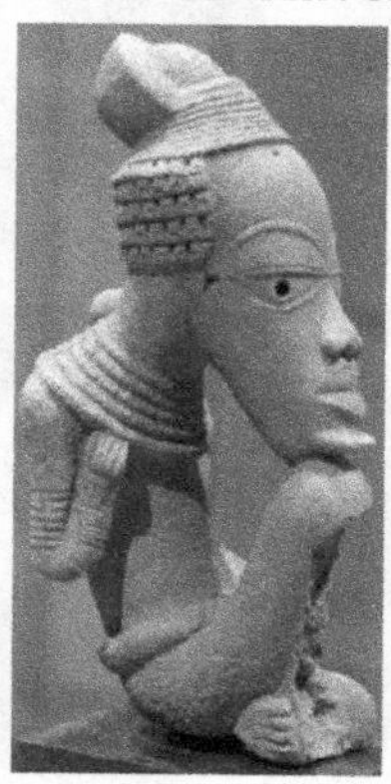

B.C which depict royal tribesman with braided hair. Our ancient Egyptian ancestors reserved braiding for royalty and for ceremonial rituals like weddings. Kings and warriors such as Tewodros I and Yamames IV who were Ethiopian emperors wore their hair in braids or cornrows dating back to the 1800s. Warriors such as those of the Masai Tribe of Kenya wear braids and cornrows even to this day. This allowed them to keep their hair clean and neat as well as out of their face in the event of battle. The Masai tribesmen also reserved this style for their rites of passage for the young men, while some of the women would shave their heads completely bald.

Additionally, our ancestors knowledge of math and geometry is expressed in the intricate styles and complicated geometric designs of hair that was parted and cornrowed into complex shapes and designs.

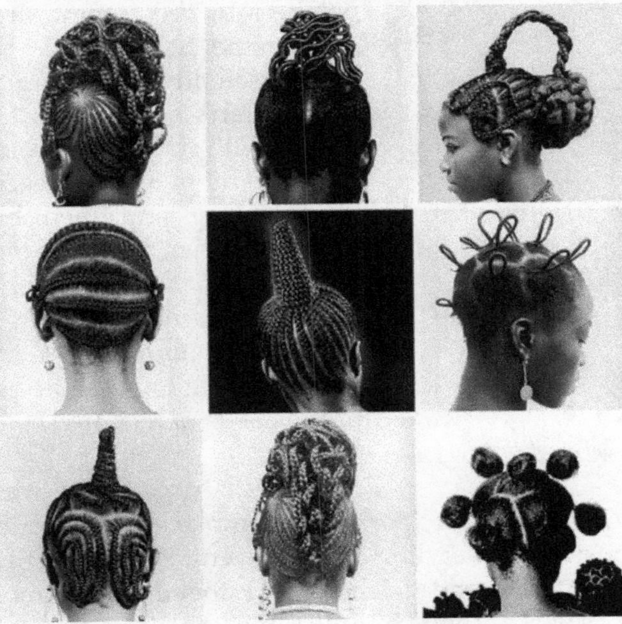

Braided styles also served as a form of communication for our ancestors. One could gather whether someone was wealthy, married, fertile, or mourning etc. Hair worn loose was not the norm. Unkempt hair was seen as someone who was not clean, or mentally unstable or mourning. This is evident in several images that we see of our African ancestors throughout the continent. Their hair is usually kept in some sort of intricate design whether it's braided, cornrowed, or even locked. It is rare to see the hair worn long and loose. If the hair is worn loose it is either partially braided, or typically worn as a short afro. Either way, having well kept and creatively designed adorned hair was a significant part of our history.

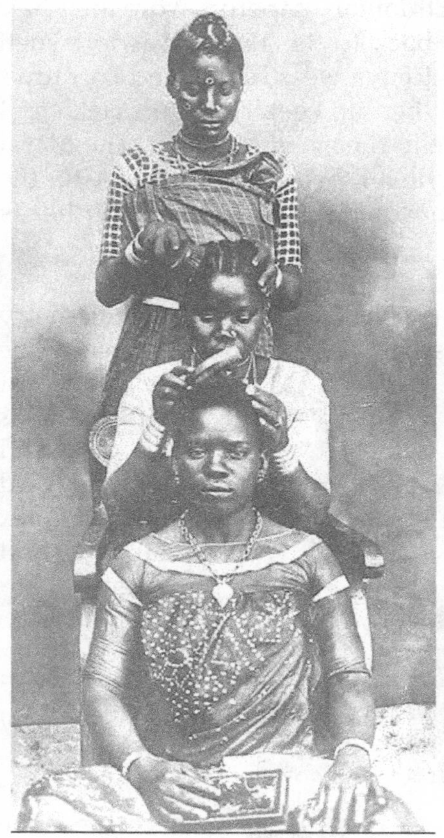

Hair groomers possessed skills to create these intricate designs. Hair grooming was considered an intimate and spiritual part of one's overall wellness. While most of us may go to hairdressers to get our hair done, traditionally our ancestor's hair stylists were family members or close members of the community. Usually the head female of the household would braid the children's hair, and teach this skill to her daughters. The daughters would learn by observing and then by doing in order to keep the craft going into the next generations. This was also done to teach the young daughters mothering skills and caring for the needs of a family.

Communal grooming was a tradition of our African ancestors. In some places, women in Africa would consider hair styling a social event. Women in the villages would commune and do their work together, braiding each others hair, as well as their children's hair. This created time for building with other sisters, where one could strengthen the bonds between each other and their roles within the community. It was not a trade as it is now, or done for a fee. Hair braiding was done for free even if it was not a family member, because even in that instance, the stylist would only be someone who the person knew closely. The women would simply do each others hair in exchange to return the favor. It was a sign of honor, confidence,

and friendship.
This is a key custom that this author encourages. Our hair is sensitive, it is our antennas and connection to the cosmos, and it carries energy. It is important for one to be conscious of who they allow to groom their hair. A hairdresser should not be haphazardly selected, they should be chosen carefully. It is recommended to select someone who we trust or have a close relationship with, because it is an intimate experience to have someone not only groom, but even touch one's hair. Similar to how our ancestors practiced, it should be considered an honor by both parties to partake in this process. Otherwise, this could result in someone not being pleased with how their hair turned out, because one may not really like or even know their hairdresser very well.

Not choosing a groomer carefully can also be the reason why one may feel completely drained of their energy, or frustrated etc.; experiencing emotions that were not their own. This is because that person's energy is now in your hair. One might find themselves wondering why they want to wash their hair out after spending half a day at the salon to get it done. So, choose your groomer carefully. A family member or trusted family friend is optimal, as well as a member of the same sex, because it helps to strengthen your sisterly or motherly bonds.

As for teenagers, if one is skilled at doing hair, they may want to limit this intimate experience to members of the same sex, or at least be cognizant of *how* they do their hair. While some of us were used to sitting between our Mother's or stylist's legs to get our hair done when we were kids, this may send the wrong or confusing message to a member of the opposite sex. We send messages through our hair, and since grooming is an intimate experience, one could possibly send mixed messages within that scenario. This is something for our young stylists to consider when choosing a member of the opposite sex as their client.

In addition, a session of hair braiding with our ancestors including shampooing, conditioning, oiling, combing, which is very similar to today. However, black soap was widely used in West and Central Africa and shea butter was also very popular and traditionally used to moisturize the hair before braiding. Combs made of natural wood were used to separate and part the hair. Overall natural products were used, there were no synthetic products put onto the hair, not even the combs.

Locs

While most people associate or trace the origins of locs to the Rastafarian movement, locs date back to our ancient African Ancestors. Our ancient Egyptian ancestors are depicted in sculptures, painting and murals wearing locs. Archeologist have discovered mummies in tombs wearing locs.

King Tut's mummy was reported as having hair that was in locs when he died. Heavily adorned plaits and locs were reserved for the extremely wealthy or royalty, therefore locs as well as braids were a symbol of power and wealth.

The Rastafarian and Locs

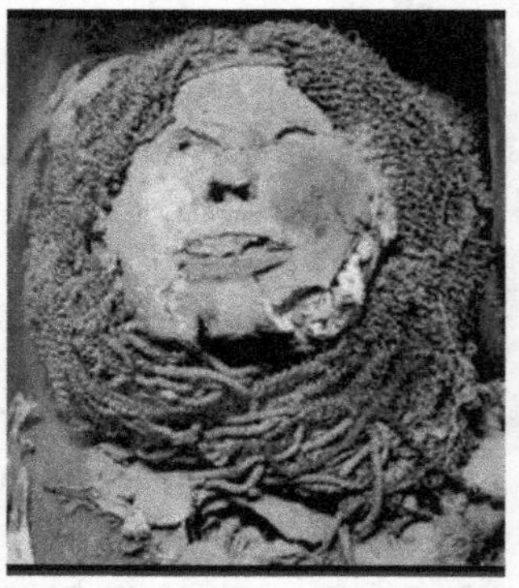

The Rastafarian Movement arose in the 1930s in Jamaica in response to their rebellions against Euro Centrism that was forced on them. At that time, Jamaica was a predominately Christian culture of which 98% were descendants of slaves. It is reported that most of them worshiped Halle Selassie I, Emperor of Ethiopia (1930s-1971). He was viewed as God incarnate or the reincarnation of Jesus. Halle Selassie was believed to be an heir of King Solomon and Queen Sheba of Ethiopia. Selassie was an Ethiopian Orthodox Christian who the Rastafarians believed would lead them into the age of prosperity and peace. The name Rastafarian comes from Haile Selassie himself. His name was Ras Tafari prior to taking the throne as Emperor of Ethiopia.

Rastafarian's locs were coined "dreadlocs" or "dreadful" by the europeans of their society who viewed them as hideous. It later evolved to the term locs which we use today. Rastafarians originally wore their hair in locs because of their Christian beliefs.

Biblically Leviticus or Numbers supported this belief which one of the tenants of the scripture requires the Nazarite followers to take several vows, one of which is to not cut their hair. They believe power and a man's strength lies in his hair, and he who chooses to cut it, gives that power away. This belief can also be referenced in the biblical story of Sampson and Delilah where Samson, a Nazarite, lost his power when Delilah cut off his 7 locs of hair. Therefore locs were reported to be a fundamental vow to be Rastafarian. To grow it, Rastas would simply not comb it, but instead wash it, twist it, and let it grow out naturally.

Some note that the Rastafarians were also inspired to wear their hair in locs when they saw a media broadcast in the 1950s of images of the Independence struggle of the feared African Mau Mau Warriors who wore locs and were seen fighting for their independence from the British Army. This hairstyle was an inspiration and served as a symbol of power and freedom from european colonizers.

Locs and Spirituality

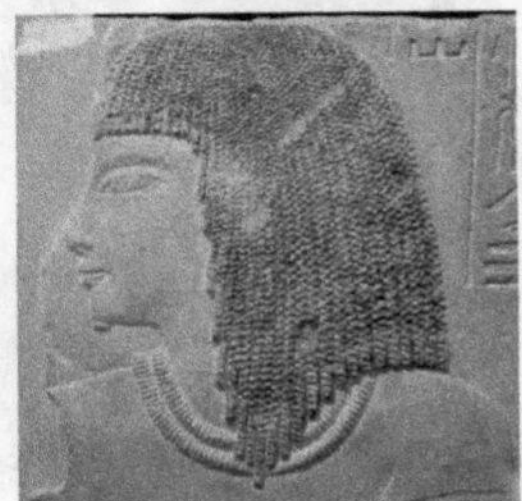

While locs originated with our African ancestors they can be referenced spiritually across several cultures.

Hinduism

In Hinduism, the Indian holy men wear locs and consider it to be a religious practice. In the myth of the Shiva deity, his full head of locs symbolize his virility and his power.

Buddhism:

In Buddhism locs can be seen to replace the traditional shaved head of their holy men. The most recognized is the Ngapas of Tibet. One of their practices is to let go of material vanity and excessive attachments. They view letting their hair grow long and freely as an expression of this belief.

Kemetic System

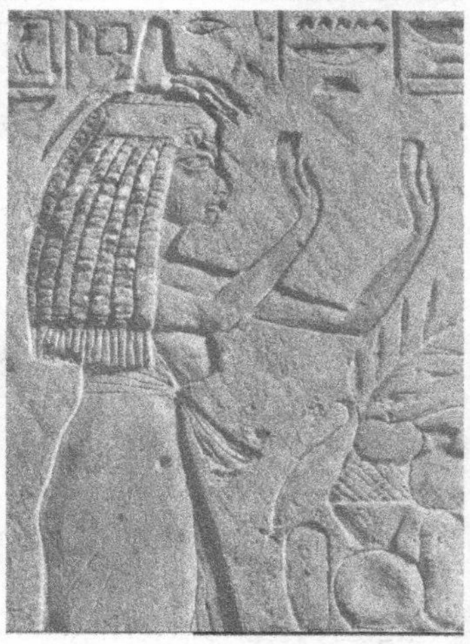

Some followers of the Kemetic system view locs as a serious matter, and that the choice to wear them should not be taken lightly. They believe locs symbolize a highly spiritual person on their journey to come closer to God. It is considered a mark of spiritual status. Some of the priests are required to wear their hair in locs while serving these Kemetic archetypes.

In general, most people associate locs with spirituality. However, the reasons are varied. It has been used as a political statement to express one's defiance or expression of their non conformity to european standards of beauty, or as a fashion statement and one's pride in their natural beauty. In many cases it does express one's commitment to some cause on some level. Locs can take years to grow long and those dedicated to that process can keep record of their commitment to their journey, whether spiritual or not, through the length of their hair.

The Afro

Last but not least we have the Afro, which got its name from the term Afro-American, and is also referred to as a natural or fro. In the late 1950 and 1960's natural hair reemerged with the presence of the Black Nationalist Movement or the Black Power Movement headed by leaders such as Marcus Garvey who spear headed the movement and opened the way for others such as Malcolm X. This called for African Americans to return to and acknowledge the truth of their roots and culture. Black Americans were encouraged to embrace hairstyles that highlighted their natural textures, and to reject the idea of using toxic chemicals such as perms to straighten the hair which identified ones alliance with the european standard of beauty which was forced on them.

This movement sparked the birth of the Civil Rights Movement which is what *specifically* associated the afro with power. We can see pictures of Angela Davis of the Black Panthers with her perfectly shaped afro and her fist in the air indicating their fight and struggle for black power. Other popular actors and actresses also wore the very large afro such as Pam Grier, The Supremes, and The Jackson 5.

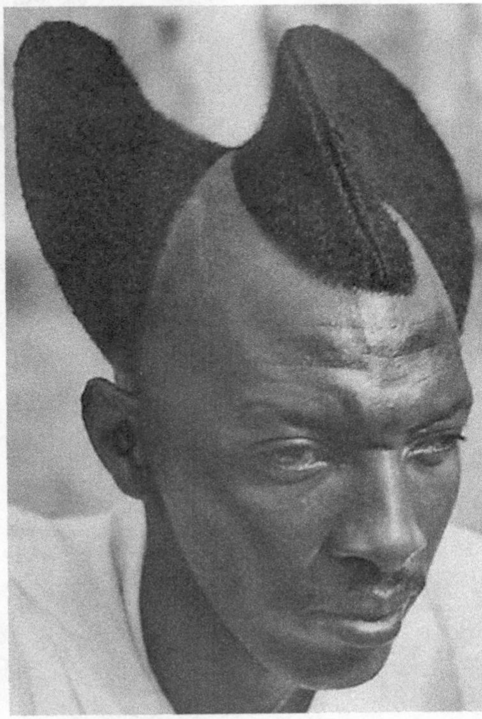

However, the afro did not originate with the black power movement. We can trace the Afro back to our very early beginnings. For many of us, the Afro is basically how our hair naturally grows out of our heads, and there are no products or chemicals needed to achieve this look.

History has shown that the popularity of the Afro, or at least the very large Afro, waned post the 1960's as it became more mainstream and was being copied by other cultures. However, present day, the Afro is coming back and not simply because of a movement, but rather because more and more people are beginning to accept and express the power of their natural beauty.

CHAPTER 5: THE HARMFUL EFFECTS OF CHEMICALS IN HAIR CARE PRODUCTS

"The very bearing of weapons changeth the mind of those that carry them."– The Forest of Life -Hindu Mythology

According to Dr. Afrika's *"Nutricide,"* there are a plethora of chemicals that are contained in relaxers which lead to various diseases and complications some of which include:

Relaxer Pre-treatment

Methylchlorol-Sothiazolimone - Alcohol that damages the liver, kidneys, nerves, and brain.

Dicetyldimonium Chloride - Poison, deadly if swallowed, used in explosives, and breaks hair. It also damages the kidneys and liver.

TEA (Triethanonlamine) - Tannic Acid, decreases blood flow to uterus and prostate.

Propylene Glycol - This ingredient is not exclusive to the perm, it is very common amongst cosmetics in general, and particularly in moisturizers, such as lotions, shampoos, and conditioners. It is marketed as a humectant and is a chemical used in antifreeze. It transports chemicals into the hair, blood, and nerves, and causes skin disease.

Polyquarternium - Poison, type of lye, and causes death if swallowed.

Relaxer Activator

Guanidine Carbonate - Holds toxic chemicals in the skin, hair, and blood.

No-Lye Relaxers

Petroleum/Mineral Oil - This is another very common ingredient in cosmetics that purports itself to be a moisturizer but it is only grease or low grade oil that actually drys the skin, clogs the pores, as well as destroys vitamins A, D, E, and K.

Calcium Hydroxide - Poison, and type of lye, used to make cement, plaster, and fireproof. It burns skin, eyes, and throat, and you can die from shock if swallowed.

PEG (Polyethylene Glycol) - Poison, destroys hair, used in anti-freeze.

Carboxylic Acid - A poison that causes high blood pressure, lung problems, and mental confusion.

Neutralizing Shampoo

Testrasodium Edta - Causes cysts, tumors, and fibroids.

Sodium Laureth Sulfate - This is another very common ingredient not exclusive to the relaxer. It is commonly found in commercial shampoos. It is a form of lye, dries the hair, prevents hair growth, and destroys and dissolves nerves, skin, bones, cells, and hair.

Disodium Cocoampho-Dipropoionate - This is used as a stain remover, and an oven cleaner. It helps chemicals to get absorbed into hair, skin, and blood.

Phenolsulfon-Phthalein – This is a form of lye, a disinfectant, machine lubricant, and it causes cancer.

Diazolidinyl Urea - This is a disinfectant that slows down the brain and nerve function, as well as causes skin irritation and convulsions, paralysis, nerve damage and cancer.

These chemicals listed were just a select few of the harmful ingredients that are contained in relaxers. This demonstrates how the product is not just localized to the hair. These chemicals get absorbed into the bloodstream and affect one's entire system. The longer they are applied the more one is at risk of having to deal with these complications, which in some rare instances can lead to death.

In addition to the hazardous conditions that can occur internally, the chemicals used in relaxers alter the hair follicle's texture and protein structure. This significantly weakens the hair causing drying, breakage, brittleness, and a lack of elasticity. Further, relaxers strip the hair of its natural oils and moisture, as well as causes irritation to the scalp which often results in lesions. While some argue that chemically straightened hair can be healthy, the very nature of this chemical process strips the hair's natural fibers of its vitality, and strength causing one's natural hair to shift from a state of health to a state of dis-ease.

Uterine Fibroids and Early Puberty

Another serious health risk associated with chemical relaxers is uterine fibroids, as well as having the ability to prematurely cause early puberty in teenage girls. There are several articles circulating regarding a study that was originally published in the "American Journal of Epidemiology." According to this article scientists followed more than 23,000 pre-menopausal Black American women from 1997 to 2009 and found that a two,to three times higher rate of fibroids amongst Black women may be linked to chemical exposure through scalp lesions and burns resulting from relaxers.

According to a separate study published in the "Annals of Epidemiology", women who got their first menstrual period before the age of 10 were also more likely to have uterine fibroids, and early menstruation which may result from hair products such as chemical relaxers.

While there is some controversy over the validity of this research, the point here is to be safer than sorry. Uterine fibroids are more common amongst Black women than any other race of women in general. It is not too far fetched to link this condition to one of our most destructive hair practices.

Uterine fibroids are noncancerous (benign) tumors that develop in the womb (uterus). However, there are severe physical complications that can result from uterine fibroids even though they are non cancerous. According to the "U.S. National Library of Medicine" some complications include:

- Severe pain or excessively heavy bleeding that may require emergency surgery.

- Twisting of the fibroid, which causes a blockage in nearby blood vessels feeding the tumor (surgery may be needed).
- Anemia (low red blood cell count) if the bleeding is very heavy.
- Urinary tract infections, if pressure from the fibroid prevents the bladder from fully emptying.
- Cancerous changes called leiomyosarcoma (rare).
- In rare cases, fibroids may cause infertility. Fibroids may also cause complications if you become pregnant, although the risk is thought to be small.
- Some pregnant women with fibroids may deliver a premature baby because there is not enough room in the womb.
- A c-section may be needed if the fibroid blocks the birth canal or causes the baby to be in a dangerous position.

The womb is a woman's life force. It is her source of creativity, and how she is fed information that she needs from the universe in order to walk within her true nature and stay connected to her highest self. It is necessary for women to honor and nurture their wombs in order to maintain their overall health, otherwise diseases will be reflected in the womb. The womb, like melanin, is very magnetic and an absorbing energy that will store toxins within its walls as a result of disregard or poor health. This can range anywhere from excessive negative thoughts (stress), synthetic foods, to drugs like chemical relaxers. While fibroids can be surgically removed, or shrunken, they usually grow back if a holistic approach is not implemented. This includes a detoxification process that involves ceasing practices that contributed to the growth of the fibroids. Choosing a healthier lifestyle, and discontinuing the use of chemical relaxers is one step closer to a healthy womb, and overall wellness.

Green Slime Found on the Brains of Black Women's Corpses

This is another topic that is circulating throughout the internet, and hair care blogs. While no one has been able to gain access to an actual autopsy report, what is interesting is that these individuals who have relatives who are coroners, or morticians, all seem to speak of a green film underneath the skin of the scalp. This film has only been found on the brains of deceased black women. The morticians and coroners deduct that it is a result of chemical relaxers. One mortician described it as a cap that flaked off the black woman's scalp.

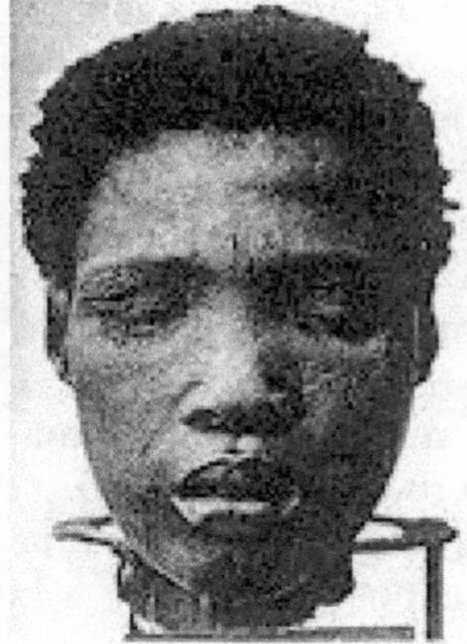
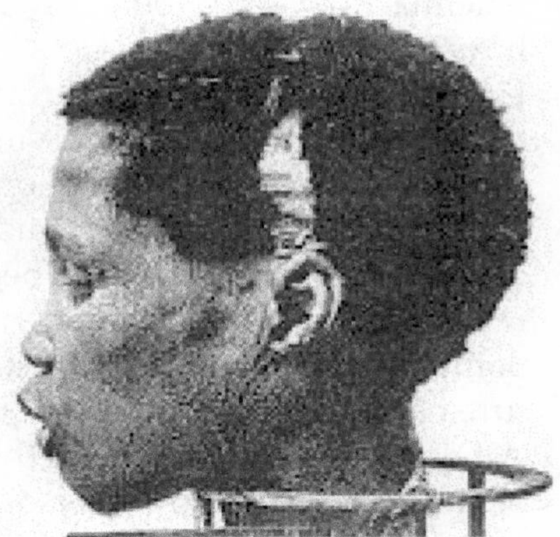

"Are our heads still being removed for experimentation?"

Without having read an actual autopsy report, this author cannot affirm that this is in fact a result of relaxing one's hair. However, it is clear that harmful chemicals that are applied to the hair get absorbed into the bloodstream through the scalp. Chemical relaxers are a common practice amongst black women, and given that the scalp is exposed to these chemicals, it is not unreasonable for one to conclude that there is a link between the green slime and hair relaxers.

The fact remains that a foreign green substance is found on the corpse of black women with relaxers, and who knows what it may have interfered with while they were alive. Chemical relaxers cause a multitude of complications, and there may be other hazards that have yet to be discovered. It is advisable to err on the side of caution and choose healthier alternatives instead of exposing oneself to such risks. If straight hair is desired this can be achieved with natural hair with the use of a blow dryer or hot comb. However, it is best if this is done by a natural hair professional. While heat is not ideal for naturally curly hair, it is a much healthier option than exposing oneself to chemicals. In this instance, the damage would be limited externally to the shaft of the hair, instead of the entire body, which is the case when using chemical straighteners.

The Truth About Lye and Government Regulation

It is safe to say that Dr. Afrika may have researched the ingredients in no-lye relaxers in particular because consumers tend to assume that a no-lye relaxer is a safe alternative to a relaxer that contains lye. However, one can see from what was explored that there are very dangerous chemicals that are contained in no-lye relaxers. Lye and no-lye products are equally dangerous; toxic is simply toxic. To say that something is "less" toxic does not take away from that fact that the nature of this product is still harmful.

The hair care industry is not regulated by the FDA. There are laws that require the hair care industry to accurately label their cosmetics, but this is not always the case. For example, according to an article titled *"Toxic Hair Treatment Highlights Need to Regulate Industry,"* published in *"Gender Across Borders,"* it uncovered that a hair smoothing treatment called the Brazilian blowout contains harmful levels of formaldehyde, which is a known carcinogen. This information came to surface where the government only stepped in because salon workers began to have nose bleeds. They also developed breathing problems which resulted from breathing in the toxic fumes all day that occur after applying heat to this formaldehyde product. Interestingly enough, the product indicated that it was *formaldehyde-free* on the label.

The article also goes on to state:
"The industry is largely in charge of regulating itself. The FDA's own website states: "Cosmetic firms are responsible for substantiating the safety of their products and ingredients before marketing."
"The Campaign for Safe Cosmetics has found black women are disproportionately affected by the lack of regulation of the beauty industry. Skin lighteners, hair straighteners — and other products designed to make women of color look more like white women — contain some of the most noxious stuff on the market, the group found. Plus, black women spend twice as much on skin care as women in other demographics, according to research cited by the group. These products and others are not regulated, meaning our bodies are being poisoned, every day, with chemicals linked to cancer and infertility."

It may appear that the solution to help protect Black women is to have the government regulate the hair care industry, but think again. The FDA is not a board of scientists who test products to ensure that they do not pose health risks to its consumers. The FDA is composed of board members of corporations and businesses whose number one priority is profit; not health. The only solution is for individuals to regulate the hair care industry by educating themselves about the ingredients contained in hair care products, and avoiding those that are laden with toxic chemicals. If one makes their health a priority, they will have no need for skin lighteners, or chemical hair straighteners, and they can also save their dollars in the process. One has to rely on themselves to implement their own preventive health care methods in order to obtain a better quality of health.

Relaxers and the Professionals

Salons that apply chemical relaxers create a harmful environment in the process. The odor that emanates from an "activated" relaxer is extremely potent. There usually is no special "relaxer room" to apply this chemical; they are generally applied by stylists out in the open in front of everyone. This leaves clientele as well as the stylist exposed to poisonous fumes that get absorbed into the lungs, and ultimately the person's entire system which exposes them to health risks.

In addition to the internal damage that occurs, external damage to the hair often results even when relaxers are applied by a professional. Many people have experienced breakage, scalp lesions, and over-processing at the hands of a professional. Further, the styling processes that accompany a perm are extremely damaging. Hot blow-dryers, or piping hot oven barrel curlers rob the hair if its moisture, and damage the structure of the hair. This process causes relaxed hair to become excessively dry, causing split ends, and a dry and brittle appearance.

Natural hair care salons are usually the best option for maintaining the health of one's hair because they specialize in natural hair, and generally use natural products. The environment is safe as well as their practices since most of them do not apply chemicals to the hair. This allows for one to maintain the health of their entire body as well as their hair.

Harmful Effects of Weaves

In an article titled *"Killed by Her Hair Extensions,"* published in *"Mail Online,"* a woman died from a massive allergic reaction, that according to the pathologist may have been caused by the glue in her hair extensions, or the solvents used to remove the glue. She collapsed in front of her doorway after coming home from a club where she had been dancing all night. The court found that the sweating from dancing may have caused glue to enter her into her blood stream.

This woman was only 34 years old, and there was no drug use reported, and according to the article she did not have any other health issues. However, it was cited that she wore weaves, and relaxers since she was 20 years old.

According to the Pathologist this allergic reaction is called anaphylactic shock, and further he states:

"I've seen cases where people using solvent to apply extensions has actually caused anaphylactic shock. There are about ten to 20 deaths a year in this country, many more in America. I have seen four in the last three months."

Anaphylaxis is a serious allergic reaction marked by swelling, hives, or lowered blood pressure. If one goes into anaphylactic shock it can become fatal if not immediately treated.

Another near fatal instance of anaphylactic shock was sighted in the media through a documentary that actress and comedian Countess Vaughn did in order to share her near death experience with this allergic reaction and her hair glue. Countess Vaughn is not only known for her talent as an actress, comedian, and singer, but she is also well known for her weaves. Starring in *"Moesha,"* and *"The Parkers,"* as well as reality TV shows, she never left home without them. Her weaves were particularly noticeable because she typically only wore blonde weaves, with light colored contact lenses to accent them.

Countess Vaughn went on to explain that her first problem with her weave occurred when she began to get lacerations on her scalp from the hair glue. The glue had not only ripped the hair, but it ripped the skin from her scalp to the point where she had to be hospitalized to treat the lacerations. Her second encounter was when she got poisoned from the chemicals used in the hair glue. While she went into anaphylactic shock, her allergic reaction did not prove to be fatal, but she shared that she did almost lose her life.

One's health or life should not be sold for a false sense of femininity or beauty. Natural beauty is healthy and priceless.

The Harmful Effects of Hair Dye

Allergic Reactions:
The ingredients in hair dye also contain chemicals that cause damage to one's hair and health. Some of the short term risks associated with hair dye are hair loss, breakage, and allergic reaction. Anaphylactic shock can also occur as a result of dying one's hair.

The key toxic ingredient that causes these allergic reactions is called PPD. PPD is also known as P-Phenylenediamine. It is an extremely noxious chemical that has been banned in some countries in Europe as well as Japan. It is the main ingredient in most commercial hair dyes and is poisonous to the immune system, as well as other major organs including the skin, nervous system, and respiratory system. Allergic reactions can occur at any time, even if one is currently exposed to, or has used the chemical in the past, therefore It is best to seek out natural alternatives.

Asthma:
Another short term effect of using hair dye is asthma. Breathing in the fumes of these chemicals on a regular basis can cause the airways to narrow, making it difficult to breathe. Studies have shown that hair stylists in particular are at extreme risk of developing asthma because they expose themselves to this chemical on a daily basis.

Cancer:
Some long term effects linked to the chemicals in hair dye, as similar to the relaxer is cancer. While some of these reports and studies are inconclusive, reports have indicated that hair dye chemicals have been proven to cause cancer in laboratory animals. However, the most evidence is in studies on hair stylists. Studies have shown that a hair stylist who has been exposed to these chemicals for more than five years has a three-times higher risk of developing cancer than one who is not exposed to these chemicals at all.

Natural Alternatives to Hair Dye

Hair in its natural state is always the healthiest. However, if one is still interested in expressing their creativity through their hair, there are in fact natural alternatives. However, my research has shown that some dyes that claim to be "natural", still contain chemicals, but claim that they are "less toxic." Again, toxic is toxic. These products should simply be avoided in general. The list of chemicals below should be taken into account to determine if the dye is truly natural. If it contains any of the ingredients below than it still contains harmful chemicals regardless of the what the label says. For instance, a "natural" hair dye company called "Naturante" has "some" natural ingredients in their hair dye products but they also contain chemicals. For this reason, they can indicate that the product is natural on their label. It is very important to read the ingredients. A rule of thumb is that if you can not pronounce it, than err on the side of caution that it may possibly be a toxic chemical. Additionally, with access to smart phones, and the internet, it only takes a few seconds to research an ingredient before you make your purchase. A product mainly consist of the first ingredients listed so those ingredients should be heavily scrutinized. This will aid one in being a responsible consumer by taking action to educate themselves about their purchases instead of relying on the hair care industry.

Below is a list of harmful chemicals to keep an eye out for that are associated with hair dye. These ingredients may be included in hair dyes that claim to be natural:

Resorcinol: A harmful irritant to the eyes and skin and is dangerous for the environment.

Ammonia: An irritant to the skin, eyes, respiratory system, and can cause asthma and breathing difficulties. This is often used as a substitute to PPD.

Persulfates: Sodium, potassium and ammonium sulfates are present in hair dyes and bleaches, and are used in concentrations of up to 60%. However, concentrations of only 17.5% have been shown to irritate skin, and persulfates are also toxic when the fumes are inhaled, causing asthma and lung damage

Lead acetate: This is present in some hair coloring products used for gradual darkening, and is another potentially toxic chemical. Lead has well-known damaging effects on the brain and nervous system.

4-ABP: This is also known as 4-Aminobiphenyl. It is used to manufacture dyes and is a known carcinogen.

Henna

Henna is a natural alternative to commercial hair dyes. It is a natural plant that grows in warm regions like Africa, and India. It is most popular for its use as art and dye on the skin. Henna is only naturally red. Any product that claims to be an all natural henna product but is not the color red has some other chemical in it. Henna will only blend with a person's current hair color. It does not lighten the hair, so to develop other hues, it has to be blended with other herbs. For instance, black can be made by blending henna and the indigo plant.

Since henna is an herb it also has healing properties. It is known to condition, cleanse and cool the scalp, as well as strengthen the hair and reduce dandruff.

One of the downsides to using henna is that it can be messy to apply and it can stain surfaces. However, it is the most natural hair dye on the market, and offers beneficial properties to the health of the hair, as well as to your physical and mental health since there are no chemical ingredients. To learn more about henna and where it can be purchased, please visit us at ***http://ihairnatural.com/ihn/black-natural-hair-type-3b/***.

Other Natural Alternatives

Lemon can be used to lighten the hair, as well as cleanse the face and scalp. The hair will lighten through exposure to the sun. This should be followed by a moisturizing conditioner as lemon is very acidic and may cause the hair to become dry and brittle.

Detoxing From The Chemicals

Transitioning Methods:

Discontinuing unhealthy practices is one of the first steps towards becoming holistically healthy, therefore embarking on a natural hair journey in an effort to detox one's system from harmful chemicals is the best decision that one can make. There are basically three methods in which one can transition back to their natural hair. However, whichever method chosen, it is advisable to wait before wearing any styles that may apply tension to the hair such as locs, or braids. It is best to be patient and allow the hair to breathe first.

After wearing chemicals for an extended period of time it will take a while for the hair to adjust back to its natural density and texture. It is recommend to wait at least six months before any big plans with one's newly natural hair. *For example, I had thin hair when I wore a perm, therefore I assumed that I would have thin natural hair. However, after months of being natural and using all natural products, accompanied by maintaining a healthy diet, my hair became very thick and dense. It was a pleasant surprise that I would not have been able to experience if I would have locked my hair immediately after returning natural.* This is the reason why some women experience thin locs, because they did not allow their hair enough time to breathe. So keep this in mind once you transition.

The Big Chop:

One very popular method is what is called "The Big Chop". As its name implies, it requires one to cut off all of their permed hair basically down to the natural roots. This method will enable one to enjoy their natural hair almost immediately, as well as allow them to enjoy a beautiful new look.

Trimming Method:

This method is done by simply trimming off the permed ends as the natural hair grows in. One can speed up the process by cutting off all of the permed ends once they achieve their desired length of natural hair. This process is not at fast as the big chop, but is more practical for those who would like to have a substantial amount of natural hair when they decided to make the full transition.

Phase Out Method

If one is not courageous enough for any type of chopping, they can do a complete grow out. This method requires patience and creativity in order to find styles that are suitable for hair that consists of two textures (natural and permed). Some women opt for this method because they do not want to cut their hair at all, particularly if it is very long. However, the longer the hair, the longer it will take for the hair to completely transition back to natural hair.

Styling Tips for Transitioners

Twist outs, braid outs, flat twists, cornrows and braids are great transitioning styles. These styles are excellent because they seamlessly blend in the two textures of permed and natural hair.

If one is in need of some inspiration for some creative ways to style their hair during this transitional period, one can go to ***iHairNatural.com*** as well as visit the style gallery in Chapter 9. There, one can find a plethora of styles for all different lengths and textures of natural hair.

Transitioning from chemical relaxers and products will begin to reverse some of the negative effects that were caused by such products. One's overall health will improve, as well as their hair and their sense of pride. One will have the ability and freedom to enjoy their hair in its natural state, and be who and what they natural are, revealing their own unique expression of their beauty and power within.

CHAPTER 6: DIETS FOR HEALTHY HAIR AND OVERALL WELLNESS

"In the Name of God, the Compassionate, the Merciful
The God of MERCY hath taught the Koran,
Hath created man,
Hath taught him articulate speech,
The Sun and the Moon have each their times,
And the plants and the trees bend in adoration.
And the Heaven, He hath reared it on high, and hath appointed the balance;
That in the balance ye should not transgress.
Weigh therefore with fairness, and scant not the balance.
And the Earth, He hath prepared it for the living tribes:
Therein are fruits, and the palms with sheathed clusters,
And the grain with its husk, and the fragrant plants.
Which then of the bounties of your Lord will ye twain deny?
He created man of clay like that of the potter.
And He created the djinn of pure fire:
Which then of the bounties, etc.
He is the Lord of the East,
He is the Lord of the West:
Which, etc.
He hath let loose the two seas which meet each other.." The Koran/Sura LV –The Merciful: 1-19

All things are connected; especially when it comes to our health, therefore a holistic approach is the best way to go in order to improve one's overall wellness. Hair and nails are last on the list to receive nutrients from our bodies. If one suffers from malnutrition it will be reflected in their hair and nails, therefore eating one type of food or vitamin will not improve one's damaged hair or health. The goal is not simply for one to focus on the health of their hair, but rather to focus on the health of their entire being.

We Require Different Foods and Medicine

In an interview titled *"Melanin,"* featuring Dr. Jewel Pookrum, MD, P.H.D. and author of *"Vitamins & Minerals from A to Z,"* Dr. Pookrum advises that since we are a melanin dominant people, we are inherently structured differently from those who are melanin deficient. Melanin requires interaction with certain amino acids, vitamins and minerals in order for it to function properly. Therefore someone who is highly melanated would require more of, as well as different types of vitamins and minerals than someone who is melanin deficient.

Dr. Pookrum further advises that due to our melanin, we have a different circulation and immune system, and our neurological awareness and how we learn is also different. Therefore, when it comes to food, it is obvious that being structurally different, we would require different foods to function at our optimal level of health. Similar to how animals are in the same mammal group; each different type of species has its own unique dietary needs. The human race is no different than this.

According to Dr. Pookrum, western medicine only truly benefits the caucasian, and as a result other races have difficulty managing their health when they use westernized standards. She advises that since we naturally have a plant based diet, we can not consume things that are biologically imbalanced such as artificial foods, as they negatively impact our melanin. Melanin will lose its capacity to cycle the energy that it is absorbing when we take in these unnatural substances. This often creates white spots in the skin of Black people who are losing their melanin as a result of poor health. It is best to maintain a holistically healthy lifestyle, and one that is measured against African centered health standards. Ethnomedicine is a sub-field of ethnobotany which is the study of the relationship between people and plants. It uses holistic measures and activates the immune system via herbs, which can be used for cleansing, detoxification, as well as to stimulate the body's self healing capabilities.

Optimal Diets for Our Health

In Dr. Llaila O. Afrika's "*African Holistic Health,*" he recommends the use of ethnomedicine, and suggests that a well balanced live food or vegetarian diet is one of the best diets for our optimal health. The following are plant based diets that are essential for our vitality:

Raw or Live Food Diet:

The "raw" or "live food" diet consists of food that is uncooked. This diet mainly consists of raw fruits, vegetables, grains, seeds, and nuts. This is one of the most advantageous diets because it is highly nutritious and consists of food that contains "life". This "life" comes in the form of enzymes that are active and alive within these foods. Foods that are cooked, canned, or contain preservatives destroy these enzymes. This is why this diet is the most optimal. Consuming live foods aid in the proper digestion and absorption of nutrients. This is often reflected in one having outstanding health, as well as a healthy outer glow and appearance. As the saying goes, "*You are what you eat.*"

Fruitarians

This diet may also fall under the umbrella of a live food or raw diet, however it solely consists of eating fruit. Seeds and nuts are also classified as fruits. Fruits are an excellent source of detoxification. They contain active enzymes which assist with digestion and the removal of toxins from the blood. These enzymes are contained in the seeds of the fruit, therefore it is essential to chew and consume the seeds while eating fruit.

According to Daniel P. Reid of "*The Tao of Health, Sex, & Longevity,*" "*It is a biological fact that fresh raw fruits and nuts contain all the vitamins, minerals, natural sugars and amino acids required for human nutrition."* However, one should consult their holistic health professional before deciding to consume a diet that solely consists of fruit. This will help one to determine if this diet is in fact suitable for their constitution, and if it will meet all of their nutritional requirements.

Vegetarian/Vegan Diets

A vegan diet may consist of both raw and cooked food. This diet does not consist of any animal products including poultry such as fish or chicken. A vegan diet also does not contain any animal by products, such as dairy products, like milk, cheese, eggs, and butter.

A vegan diet is technically a "vegetarian" diet because it consists of eating vegetation. However, this distinction between vegan and vegetarian emerged because people who consider themselves "vegetarian" may also eat fish, or animal by products such as dairy, while "vegans" do not eat any form of animal products. While this is not a text book definition of a "vegetarian", this group of people refer to themselves as such because the majority of their diet consists of vegetation. They also do not eat the flesh of land animals. This is an excellent alternative to explore for those who are looking to pace themselves into transitioning to a healthier diet.

Tips for Transitioning to a Healthier Diet

While these are some healthier dietary options to explore, one is not expected to adhere to any of them overnight. *I will share with you the guidance that I received from a loved one which allowed me to transition to a vegan diet. His advise was to continue eating according to my present diet, but to simply begin implementing the healthier foods into the diet. It sounded counterproductive but it actually worked. I no longer had cravings for certain foods, and I had eventually eliminated certain foods from my diet without even realizing it. It was not a painful, or unrealistic experience. I was able to fully transition into a healthier lifestyle with relative ease, and minimal cravings.*

This is a journey that one can embark on with a friend. I did this with a friend, and it was fun to share the results of our vegetarian and vegan recipes. We also enjoyed meeting occasionally to dine out in an effort to try different types of ethnic vegetarian dishes. This helped us to see that just because we were eating healthier; we weren't missing out on amazingly delicious cuisine. We learned that some vegans and vegetarians basically enjoy some of the same types of food as meat eaters, however a vegan's diet is much healthier. This became an eye opening experience where we enjoyed delicious meals, and desserts, as well as the improvement of our overall health.

Healthy Foods for Healthy Hair

Water:

Water is essential for one's optimal health. In addition to removing toxins from one's system and keeping it hydrated it is responsible for carrying out various functions within the body. Water assists with:

- Dissolving minerals and nutrients to make them accessible as food for the cells.
- Carrying oxygen and nutrients to cells.
- Regulating body temperature.
- Lubricating joints.
- Moistening tissues surrounding the eyes, mouth, and nose.
- Preventing constipation.
- Removing pressure from the liver and kidneys by helping to remove toxins from the body.
- Protecting the body's organs and tissues.

Our bodies consists of more than 80% water; a lack of an adequate intake can lead to various illness and diseases, including dry and brittle hair. For this reason, it is imperative that one monitors their daily intake. The recommended intake is half of one's body weight in ounces, or half a gallon to a gallon a day, if possible.

It is best to drink water at room temperature. Ice cold water with a meal can inhibit digestion because the water freezes the ducts needed to digest the food. This will cause the food to ferment or rot within the stomach resulting in gas and constipation. Scheduling consumption before or after a meal is recommended. This will prevent one from impeding digestion, as well as create more space in their stomach to receive the water.

Fruits

Most fruits are excellent for the health of one's hair because they are primarily composed of water and contain an abundance of vitamins and minerals. They are excellent cleansers as well. Fruits aid in digestion and the proper removal of waste and toxins. This prevents these toxins from being released onto the face and skin. A rule of thumb is that foods that are generally good for the skin are usually also good for the hair, since it is attached to the scalp. Further, fruits are most beneficial when eaten alone. Incompatible combinations such as with starch and proteins can impede digestion, causing food to ferment within the stomach. The seeds of fruits should also be consumed as they contain the active enzymes which assist with the absorption of nutrients and proper digestion.

Apples:

Apples are rich in vitamins and minerals including vitamins A, B, C, E, and biotin, calcium, iron, silicon, as well as sulfur. Apples are also wonderful cleansers as they aid in the removal of toxins to help maintain a healthy system, clear skin, as well as healthy hair. Additionally the sulfur in apples provides smooth skin, shiny hair, and strong nails. Other foods rich in sulfur include, onions, asparagus, and lettuce.

Cherries:

Cherries contain high levels of antioxidants, and are high in vitamins A and C. They are excellent cleansers, as they are often used as the only meal body detoxes. Cherries assist with cleaning the blood, liver, kidneys, as well as the intestines.

Grapes:

Grapes are another fruit that is an excellent cleanser of the blood, as well as the liver. Grapes contain vitamins A, B, C, iron, calcium, silicon and sulfur which is good for the skin and hair. According to Dr. Jewel Pookrum, in *"Vitamins & Minerals from A to Z"*, grapes are also one of the foods that are essential for proper melanin function, along with bananas, mushrooms, leafy greens, and vegetables.

Blueberries:
Blueberries have the most antioxidants of 40 commonly eaten fruits. They are rich in vitamin C, iron, and calcium. They are also good for cleaning the blood, and aid in the proper elimination of wastes promoting healthy hair and skin.

Blackberries:
Blackberries are rich in calcium, vitamin C, and iron. They also include minerals such as potassium, phosphorus, and sulfur which promotes healthy and shiny hair. They also aid in cleaning the blood and the intestines.

Cucumbers:
Cucumbers are rich in sulfur, potassium, sodium, silicon, and are potent diuretics. They aid in the removal of waste through the kidneys, so that these toxins will not be purged onto the face or skin. High Priest Kwatamani, author of *"Raw and Living Foods"* attributes the long hair in his family to the cucumber. Kwatamani also juices the cucumber and uses it to wash his hair which serves as a refreshing cleanser to the scalp.

Pears:
Pears are another fruit that is an excellent diuretic, as they primarily consist of water. Pears remove waste through the kidneys, and they also contain sulfur, calcium, iron, and significant amounts of vitamins A, B, and C.

Cranberries:
Cranberries are rich in vitamins A, B, and C, as well as sulfur. They are good for cleaning the kidneys and liver. Cherries promote clear skin and healthy hair.

Bell Peppers:
Bell peppers are great for clearing the skin, and are good for the hair and nails as well. They are rich in vitamin C, silicon, as well as calcium, iron, and potassium.

Dark Leafy Greens and Vegetables:

Dark leafy greens and vegetables are essential for melanin function including spinach, broccoli, swiss chard, and kale. They contain a great source of vitamin A and C which help to produce sebum which is the oil that the scalp naturally produces. Dark leafy greens are also a good source of iron and calcium.

Beans:
Beans and legumes such as kidney beans and lentils should be an important part of one's hair care diet. They provide plentiful protein to promote hair growth, and ample iron, zinc, and biotin. Biotin is necessary for proper immune function. A deficiency can cause a myriad of problems including skin disorders as well as hair loss.

Nuts:
Nuts such as brazil nuts are one of nature's best sources of selenium which is an important mineral for the health of the scalp. Walnuts contain alpha-linolenic acid, and omega-3 fatty acids that help to condition the hair. They are also good sources of zinc; as are cashews, pecans, and almonds. A zinc deficiency can lead to hair shedding

Wheat Germ:
Wheat germ is rich in silicon, which builds strong fingernails, and healthy hair. It is also good for the skin. It helps with the digestion of fats and the elimination of wastes preventing eruptions on the surface of the skin.

Exercise

This chapter would not be complete without a discussion about exercise. Exercise is essential for maintaining one's health, and it is one of the most overlooked components to one's hair care regimen. It keeps us healthy and strong, and prevents stagnation. It also aids in the removal of toxins and waste from the body.

Exercise releases endorphins which gives one a sense of well-being, and this helps to reduce stress which is one of the main causes of hair loss. A stressful event can prematurely force hair follicles into the telogen phase of their life cycle. This causes excessive shedding and thinning of the hair.

However, some forms of exercise can actually be stressful on the body, particularly westernized exercises such as running or weight lifting that can tighten, and tense the body. This usually leads to injury.

Below are some forms of exercise that consist of stretching and rhythmic movements, leaving one feeling refreshed instead of depleted of their energy.

Breathing:
Breathing is a form of exercise. Inhaling extracts the negative ions from the air which provide the body with energy and nutrition. The upward and downward movement of the diaphragm massages the body's organs improving their vitality. It also promotes healthy circulation of blood and oxygen within the system as well.

Yoga:
Yoga is traditionally a form of spirituality, however in modern day practices it is commonly seen as a form of exercise, or a combination of both. Yoga is excellent because it consists of natural flowing movements that are lead by the breath. This movement helps to remove blockages, and circulate oxygen throughout one's system. It also reduces stress, releases toxins, improves posture, and increases flexibility. Certain postures such as "downward facing dog" or "the wheel" stimulate hair growth due to their ability to circulate blood to the scalp.

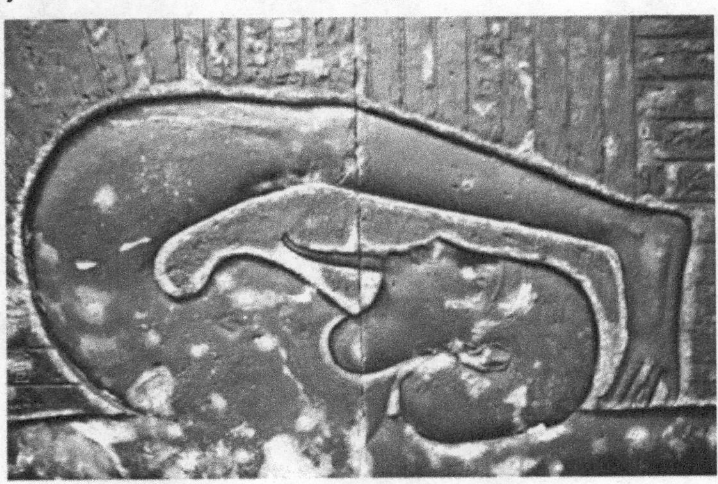

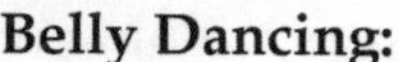

Belly Dancing:

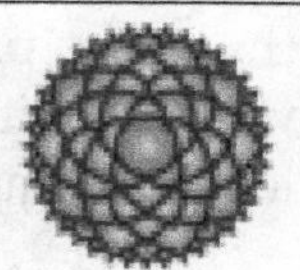

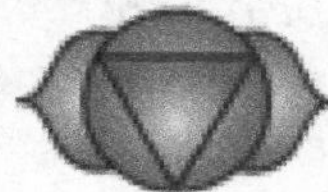

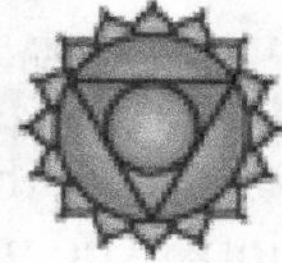

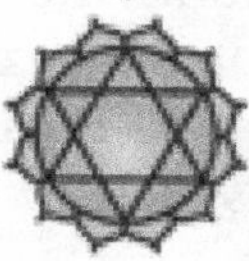

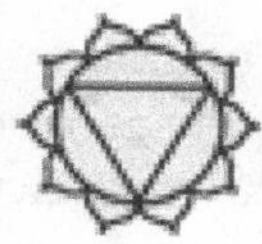

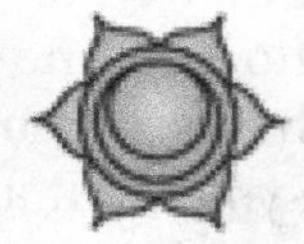

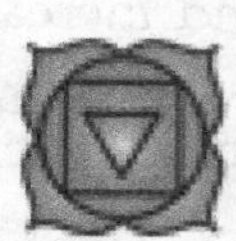

Belly dancing is also a fantastic form of exercise. It consists of controlled breathing and rhythmic movements that shift and balance energy throughout one's body. It also tones muscles and massages the organs. Belly dancing aids in balancing the chakras. The chakras are focal points on our spiritual bodies that receive and transmit energy, and govern one's emotional and physical state. A regular routine will improve one's emotional well-being and their overall wellness.

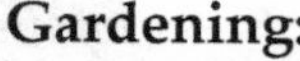

Gardening:

Activities such as gardening are also a great way to exercise. Weeding, and planting flowers and vegetables work the muscles in the arms and legs. It also gives one exposure to the elements since it is conducted outdoors. Gardening is an excellent way to stay connected to the earth, which is another reflection of our femininity. The soil aids in drawing out the toxins from the body through the feet. It is best done with bare feet and bare hands where possible. This is also another way in which our women are fed information from nature. We receive it from the earth through our wombs. For this reason, gardening, particularly, is an exercise of choice.

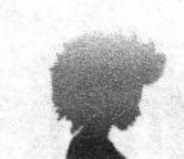

CHAPTER 7: NATURAL HAIR MAINTENANCE

"Pansa Oju ina a baa dudu petepete
Blackened calabash food receptacle above the fire place
Obun lo t ok obo lo ri siasia
A dirty person returns from the farm looking more filthy"
– Ose-Otura (Gaining Power)-
The Sacred Odu Ifa

The Newly Natural

When most women or young ladies transition back to their natural hair, they are initially filled with questions and concerns regarding their newly natural hair. Some even second guess their decision to go natural and return back to the chemicals. There are generally three reasons why this may occur:

1. Difficulty excepting what one looks like with their newly natural hair.

2. The person did not take the necessary time that is required to let their hair breathe so that their true texture and density and can fully grow in.

3. The person did not take the time to research how to manage natural hair as well as their specific texture.

The Adjustment Phase

This is what this author calls "the adjustment phase" which is slightly different from the transitioning phase. This phase occurs over the very first few days/weeks of returning natural. During this time one may be at a loss with what to do with their unfamiliar hair, as well as unsure of if they even like it. This author suggests that during this time one arm themselves with the three tools below:

1. The ability to see oneself with new eyes.

2. Patience.

3. Love and tenderness towards one's hair including thorough research and education on how to manage natural hair.

Item #1 has been covered all throughout this book. However, if one is still struggling with this concept, this author suggests that one look at themselves in the mirror on a daily basis to get accustomed to seeing themselves in their natural state. *Run your fingers through your hair daily to get familiar with your curls and texture.*

Talk to your hair. Just as similar to talking to plants or flowers, natural hair is alive and will be receptive to the love that you are sending it. Tell your hair how much you love it. Even apologize to it for hiding or altering its natural beauty under chemicals and weaves. Next, listen to your hair. It will guide you as to what it likes and does not like. This will help one to have a healthy interactive relationship with their hair, and they will be amazed at how well their hair responds.

Item #2 is certainly required in this phase, as well as all throughout one's natural hair journey. It will take time to figure out what styles, as well as what products work best for one's hair. It may also take some time if one may have goals for growing long natural hair, therefore patience is required. This is the time to let the hair simply breathe in order to allow it to return to its true texture and density. This will result through healthy diet, exercise, and a healthy hair care regimen. It is best not to overwhelm one's hair in this phase with stressful styles or an over abundance of products. An Afro style is optimal during this time as well as a low maintenance hair care regimen.

Item #3 is also covered throughout this book and is required in order to maintain a healthy relationship with one's hair. Further, education is the first step to building a proper hair care and maintenance regimen.

Washing

While washing is an obvious component of any hair care regimen this step is usually not done properly. Hair should always be clean; hair that is not clean can be unsightly and stunt growth. Unclean hair results from exposure to one's environment, product buildup, and inconsistent washing. A washing schedule should be created in order to prevent product buildup and clogged pores on the scalp. For some that is once a week, once a month, or even daily depending on one's hair type, environment, diet, and lifestyle.

When to Wash

If one listens to the signals that their hair is sending them, they will be able to determine a proper washing schedule. Itchy scalp is a sign of product buildup and a clear indication that it is time to wash one's hair. It is best if the hair is washed once per session instead of two or three times that some may be accustomed to. Excessive washing in a single session can dry the hair out even when using a moisturizing shampoo. One thorough wash on a weekly basis is an ideal schedule. This will keep the hair clean and manageable since it is not stripped of its natural oils. However, if one is in need of a deep cleaning, a clarifying shampoo once a month is recommended. This should be used moderately and followed up with a moisturizing shampoo in order to maintain an adequate moisture balance.

How to Wash

Hair should be washed in the direction of the hair cuticle which is downwards, similar to how it is done at hair salons. This will help to prevent tangles and ensure that the cuticle lies flat which will prevent moisture loss, and give the hair a shiny appearance. It is also important to be careful to not scratch the scalp when washing one's hair. The scalp should be massaged using the tips of the fingers. This helps to stimulate the scalp and promote hair growth. One should also refrain from using an excessive amount of shampoo during a wash session. This will cause the hair to become dry and create product buildup if not thoroughly rinsed. A small amount should suffice and provide a sufficient lather to cleanse the hair.

Pre-Poo

A pre-poo is a treatment applied prior to shampooing that may consist of moisturizers, oils and/or conditioners. Most women tend to use their favorite conditioners or create a blend of their favorite oils. A pre-poo is usually done in order to prevent moisture loss during the shampoo process which can be drying depending on how often one washes their hair or the shampoo being used.

Pre-poos are beneficial in reducing hygral fatigue, which is the expanding and contracting of hair as water enters and exits. For this reason, this process is believed to help protect the cortex and cuticle of the hair.

Pre-poos are like pre-deep conditioning treatments that most people find beneficial. This method helps to keep the hair detangled during the washing process, which results in less breakage. It also helps to keep the hair soft and moisturized after washing.

Co-Washing

Co-Washing is the method of using a conditioner to wash the hair in replace of using a shampoo. This is an excellent option for tightly coiled black natural hair which has a tendency to become dry. Using a conditioner instead of a shampoo will limit exposure to harsh cleansing agents such as sulfates which strip the hair of its natural oils. This method helps to maintain the hair's proper moisture balance which is essential for natural kinky and curly hair. However, some commercial conditioners contain sulfates so it is best to be careful and read the ingredients. Further, depending on how much product is used on one's hair, this method may result in product build up since conditioners contain agents that are deposited onto the hair, instead of lifting or removing build up from the hair. For this reason, it is best to alternate between washing with both a shampoo and conditioner as needed.

Shampoos to Avoid

Commercial shampoos, particularly those marketed towards people with straight hair should be avoided because they contain harsh cleansing agents as well as toxic ingredients. These shampoos are not suited for black natural hair. Straight hair tends to hold more oil because the scalp's natural oil (sebum) can easily penetrate the entire shaft of straight hair. Shampoos for straight hair strip black natural hair of its moisture. This can cause black natural hair to become dry, dull, and brittle which leads to breakage.

Many commercial products geared towards African Americans are not necessarily owned by them. Some of these products may not be as natural as they purport to be, and may contain some of the same harsh chemicals that are found in shampoos geared towards people with straight hair. Please re-examine Chapter 5 to identify some of the toxic ingredients that should be avoided. Some other ingredients include:

- **Sulfates-** Sulfates are salts of sulfuric acid used in personal care products as cleansing agents. They strip hair of its moisture causing drying and breakage.
- **Parabens-** Parabens are chemicals used as preservatives in personal care products. They can cause allergic reactions and irritate the skin. They have also been linked to breast cancer due to their ability to mimic estrogen which causes tumors to grow.
- **Silicones-** Silicones are synthetic compounds that are also used in personal care products. They are lubricants that coat the hair similar to grease. They repel water causing the hair to become dry due to the loss of moisture.
- **Alcohol** - Alcohol in its purest form is extremely drying on the hair. Some alcohols are emulsifiers that can be derived from vegetable sources such as cetearyl alcohol. However, it is important to check the ingredients as most emulsifiers are derived from animal fats which may be problematic for those with vegetarian diets. If it is derived from natural sources it will indicate "vegetarian" or "derived from vegetable sources" on the label.

Natural ingredients can also prove to be problematic for someone with allergies to natural foods such as wheat or nuts. It is important to reference the ingredients in one's personal care products in order to prevent allergic reactions or the use of toxic or undesired ingredients in general.

How to Read Ingredients

The ingredients within a product are listed in the order of their quantity. If a product's label includes "olive oil" but it is one of the last ingredients listed, then this product contains very little olive oil if any at all. If water or natural ingredients and oils are not listed first then it is probably a low quality product. Ingredients determine the quality of a product, not its label or price. There are some higher quality products that may not contain all natural ingredients. However, for those that are seeking 100% natural products I will share the sound advice that was passed down to me when it comes to selecting personal care products.

"If you can't eat it, don't put it on your skin or hair."

Problems Related to Unclean Hair

Acne breakouts

Acne breakouts have been associated with unclean hair. This has been linked to longer hair in particular when the oils and products from the hair touch the skin on the face. This causes the face to become oily, clogs pores and creates breakouts. This can also result from the face rubbing against a pillow that is saturated with hair oil. This is often the case for those who do not cover their hair when they sleep at night.

Hair Loss

Unclean hair can also lead to hair loss. In cases of extreme buildup of oil and dirt, the hair follicles are not getting the oxygen that it needs in order to continue to grow. Hair that is not washed regularly or left untouched can cause matting. Matting of the hair leads to hair loss, as the removal of the matting often results in shedding, or one having to cut out large patches of hair.

Headaches

Studies have shown that some people get tight scalp or severe headaches when they do not wash their hair for a long period of time. Tight scalp is caused because the sebum and product buildup cakes up on the scalp to the point where the scalp can not move or breathe. This creates tightness of the scalp which can result in headaches.

Dandruff

Dandruff is not only limited to dry hair. It is also caused by a fungus called malassezia which feeds on natural oils. It is more prone to grow rapidly on hair that is dirty in general as opposed to hair that is simply dry. In extreme cases it can cause hair loss. Treatment for this is regular washing or in severe cases, medicated shampoos.

Conditioning

Conditioning helps to restore moisture that is loss during the washing process. It also restores elasticity, increases shine, prevents breakage, and increases manageability. There are several types of conditioners on the market, such as leave-ins, instant, and deep conditioners. Whichever one is chosen, it is important to read the ingredients and follow the instructions provided on the label. Some ingredients like peppermint or tea tree oil can be used to stimulate the scalp which improves circulation and promotes hair growth. Water should also be the first ingredients listed. This will ensure that the product contains an ample amount of moisture.

While moisture is paramount to the health of black natural hair, selecting a conditioner that also contains protein is important. Hair is made up of over 80% protein. Applying protein to the hair will aid in keeping the hair strong, provide elasticity, and maintain a proper moisture and protein balance.

Deep Conditioning

Deep conditioning helps the hair to become more manageable and can assist with softening hair texture where manageability is an issue. This is especially the case if this is done on a routine basis; particularly after every wash. If heat is applied this process can help to soften the hair. The heat will open up the cuticle to allow a deep penetration of moisture to be delivered to the cortex of the hair. For this reason, deep conditioning can be done with any type of conditioner when heat is applied. This can be done with the use of a plastic cap and a hooded dryer set on medium heat. If one does not have access to a hooded dryer they can wrap a towel around their plastic cap and let it sit for at least 30 minutes. At least 15-30 minutes of warm heat is required with both methods to allow the moisture to penetrate the cortex of the hair.

How to Apply Conditioner

While the hair is still wet it should be sectioned off into at least four parts. The hair should be detangled with fingers or a comb by gently removing the tangles working from the bottom of the strand up. This helps to minimize breakage. Once the section is completely detangled one can use their finger or a fine tooth comb to apply conditioner to that section. Next, put in a loose twist to keep the hair out of the way and move on to the next section of hair. Repeat this process all throughout the hair. This process will ensure that every strand of hair gets conditioned, and that tangles are gently removed which will help to retain hair length.

Over Conditioning and Protein

It is possible to over condition one's hair. This is generally the case if one uses a conditioner that is not balanced with an adequate amount of protein. Symptoms of over conditioned hair include hair that is too soft, weak or limp. If a protein conditioner is not desirable, one can supplement their hair care regimen with a protein treatment at least once a month.

A natural protein treatment that was recommended to me by a loved one was to use eggs. This can be accomplished by cracking open an egg and mixing it with a natural oil and lightly warming this mixture on the stove. A warm temperature will prevent the egg from cooking. Next, apply the mixture to the hair. If one desires a deep treatment, a plastic cap and towel is suggested instead of a hooded dryer. This will ensure that the egg does not cook on the hair and serve as a nice deep conditioning protein treatment.

Moisturizing

Moisture consists of condensed or diffused liquid; especially water. Water is the most optimal form of moisture as it contains oxygen and water. However, due to its ability to quickly evaporate, moisturizers that contain water and other ingredients like humectants and natural oils are more preferred options for moisturizing one's hair. Humectants such as vegetable glycerin, honey, or aloe vera are wonderful ingredients because they absorb moisture from the air and attach it to itself. This helps to prevent moisture loss. Despite this fact, if humectants are used in arid environments, this can cause the hair to become dry because they will absorb moisture from one's hair since it can not absorb it from the air.

Products such as grease and oils are not moisturizers. Grease is a form of mineral oil or petroleum that simply coats the hair and clogs pores. While natural oils lubricate the hair and deliver their medicinal benefits to the hair, since they do not contain water, they do not provide moisture. However, they are excellent options for sealing in moisture which is why they are generally applied to wet hair after it has been conditioned or moisturized.

Moisturizers can be applied to the hair as needed. This can be done daily, or whenever the hair begins to feel dry, as long as enough is used to replenish the moisture content of the hair.

How to Dry Natural Hair

While there are certain products or natural styles that require blow drying or hot combing, using appliances that emit heat at unusually high temperatures is not beneficial to black natural hair. This type of heat depletes hair of its moisture and damages the outer layer of the hair shaft. It is highly recommend to air dry black natural hair in order to prevent moisture loss. Frequent use of heat can also cause the hair to lose its natural texture and curl pattern. If this happens, one has to get their hair cut off in order to restore it back to its natural state. Most common natural hair styles can be set and air dried. However, if one desires a style that requires heat they should consult a natural hair care professional that specializes in using heat or straightening natural hair.

Trimming

Trimming the ends of ones hair helps to give the hair a much neater appearance. However, contrary to popular belief; it does not make hair grow longer, therefore a trimming schedule is not required. One can trim their hair on an as needed basis. One technique that can be used is called "dusting." This is done by sectioning off the hair into little twists after it has been washed or conditioned. Next, cut off the small tips of each twist where the ends appear to be split. This process allows one to remove split ends without altering the shape of their hair. Otherwise, if one is interested in getting their hair shaped, or cut into a particular style, it is recommended to seek out a natural hair stylist that is skilled in cutting natural hair. This will help one to determine what shape is most suitable for their face and texture.

Protecting Your Crown

Hair Wrapping

While this author encourages the revealing of one's crown, it is also beneficial to occasionally give the hair a rest, and protection by covering it. Black natural hair is alive. It serves as a conductor for receiving as well as transmitting energy; positive and negative. This is sometimes one of the reasons why people cut their hair off because they feel heavy with the energy that is surrounding it. This is often the case for those who wear locs. Since they do not cut their hair often they will have the same hair on their heads for years or decades, in some cases.

If one is not interested in doing a series of big chops throughout their natural hair journey, hair wrapping is an excellent alternative. One can use beautiful scarves or fabrics to wrap their hair. They come in various shapes, colors, sizes, and designs. If one is in need of inspiration please visit our site at ***www.ihairnatural.com*** to learn more. Covering will protect one's crown from receiving harmful energy that one may interact with on a daily basis. This allows one to be grounded, and think clearly since they are not constantly picking up unwanted or negative energy.

Smudging

This is a wonderful alternative for protecting or spiritually cleansing one's crown, especially if one is not interested in big chops or covering their hair. Smudging is simply the process of taking an herb such as sage, or any natural element that you can burn such a dried leaves, or tree resin like myrrh, and lighting it with fire on a charcoal disc or incense burner. This will create a smoke that you will then use to "smudge" out your hair as a form of cleansing and removal of any negative energy. During this process, you can also affirm or state what it is that you want cleansed from your hair, as well as any affirmations or desires that you want to fortify your hair with. Usually there will be enough smoke where you can smudge your entire body in the process giving yourself a full body spiritual cleanse. To learn more about how to smudge hair, please come visit us at *www.ihairnatural.com*.

Bedtime Routine

There are several methods for which one can choose to protect their hair at night. Some women who wear twist outs will re-twist their hair every night and cover it with a silk scarf or bonnet. Another method is to leave the hair out and sleep on a silk pillow instead. This is ideal because it eliminates the need to constantly manipulate the hair. Too much manipulation on dry natural hair can lead to breakage. Another option is to simply cover the style with a silk scarf and re-fluff the style in the morning.

This technique is similar to was is called "pineappling". This serves well, in particular, for Afro styles such as twist or braid outs where a scarf would be too restricting and completely flatten out the hair style. Pineappling is more of a softer hold. The curls are molded upwards like the shape of a pineapple, and silk or satin fabric is used to wrapped around the hair which is secured with a pin. In the morning, one can simply take down their wrap and re-fluff their curls.

Whatever bedtime routine is selected it is beneficial to apply moisture to the hair at night. This will provide the hair with additional protection by preventing moisture loss throughout the night.

How to Grow Long Natural Hair

Many naturals are interested in learning the "secret" to growing long natural hair, unfortunately there is no special secret or a single special product that will help one to grow it. While black natural hair grows about 6 inches a year on average, the rate of growth can depend on various factors such as genetics, environment, curl pattern, and one's overall health. The good news is that if one implements the hair maintenance techniques that have been suggested, and develops their own healthy practices, accompanied with a healthy lifestyle, one will certainly have no trouble achieving length and maintaining a healthy head of natural hair.

Keeping a simple hair care regimen and implementing low manipulation practices such as protective styling will assist with this goal. The less one bothers their hair, the more it will grow. Think of women who have beautiful locs flowing way down past their shoulders. The key is that they do very little to their hair. There is little manipulation or products involved, and they wash and moisturize their hair on a routine basis. Maintaining these healthy practices, and the health of one's mind, body and spirit will certainly be reflected in the beauty of their crown.

CHAPTER 8: NATURAL HAIR TEXTURE/TYPES & PRODUCTS

"You have many good qualities and have rendered great service, but you must always remember not to become conceited. You are respected by all, and quite rightly, but this easily leads to conceit. If you become conceited, if you are not modest and cease to exert yourselves, and if you do not respect others, do not respect the cadres and the masses, then you will cease to be heroes and models. There have been such people in the past, and I hope you will not follow their example."

–Chairman Mao Tse-Tung

Natural black hair comes in an array of different textures. Understanding the nature of one's *unique* texture is fundamental to learning how to care for it. However, healthy natural hair in general should exhibit traits of high elasticity, strength, shine and low to normal porosity.

Hair Porosity

"Porous hair", is a term used to describe how well the hair shaft and its cortex is able to be penetrated by water or chemicals. There are three levels of porosity.

Low Porosity: Low porosity is used to describe hair that has very tightly bound cuticle layers where the individual cuticle scales lie flat and overlap one another. This results in hair that is very shiny, especially if it is dark in color. Overall this type of hair is considered to be quite healthy. If one has hair that repels water then it is a good indication that it has low porosity. This type of hair is also described as being quite difficult to process because it resists the penetration of chemicals.

Normal Porosity: Hair possessing average or normal porosity will be relatively easier to maintain because it allows moisture to pass into the cortex as needed, but resists permitting too much water to penetrate it. Normal porosity hair also has a tendency to hold styles better.

High Porosity: Highly porous hair is the result of damage to the hair shaft through the use of chemical processes, harsh treatments, and environmental exposure. This damage creates gaps and holes on the surface of the hair shaft. In general, highly porous hair has characteristics of being dry no matter how much moisturizer or conditioner is added to it. This occurs because moisture is loss through the exposed cuticle layer that will not lie flat and seal in the moisture that is added to the hair. Since the cuticle is open it will absorb moisture easily, but, also lose the moisture just as easily. Some symptoms of highly porous hair include:

• Hair that is very moist when wet, but has lost all of its moisture once it has dried
• Hair that dries very quickly
• Hair that tends to process chemicals like relaxers very quickly

Hair Porosity Test:

Another way to test hair porosity is to test whether or not it floats in water. If the hair floats in water, then this is evidence of a healthy cuticle. The hair floats because it does not have any gaps in its cuticle. Highly porous hair will sink because it will soak up all of the water due to the raised cuticle and gaps along the hair shaft.

Treatment for Highly Porous Hair:

Cutting off the Damaged Hair: If the hair is highly damaged from chemical processing and thermal treatment, the damaged hair may need to be cut. Some damage to the cuticle layer may be reparable but only to a certain extent.

Apple Cider Vinegar Rinse:

An Apple Cider Vinegar rinse is recommend for highly porous hair. It is so widely used that it is referred to by its acronym ACV. It is also used by those with normal to low porosity hair as a maintenance treatment to help seal in moisture and retain shine. Other products that cater to highly porous hair may be marketed as conditioners for "color treated hair" because they are usually on the acidic side. Apple Cider Vinegar is also mildly acidic, and a cheaper alternative to some pricey conditioners.

Apple Cider Vinegar temporarily constricts the cuticles correcting porosity levels. For those with highly porous hair, it is recommended to do an ACV rinse on a weekly basis. This can be reduced once the cuticle is repaired.

Apple Cider Vinegar can be purchased in a local supermarket and on our website at: ***http://ihairnatural.com/ihn/hair-care-regimens/natural-hair-growth/***, and a little goes a long way. One can take ¼ of a cup or less and added it to 2 to 3 cups of water. This mixture can be placed into a spray bottle and used as a final rinse (do not rinse out). This will help one's hair to become shinier and tangle free, allowing the cuticle to lie flat reflecting the rays and light of the sun.

Cold Water Rinse:

A cold water rinse is another method that can be used to flatten hair cuticles. This is an excellent option after a moisturizer or deep conditioning treatment has been applied to the hair. Heat allows the cuticle to swell open so that moisture can be delivered to the cortex of the hair. Cold temperatures like cold water close the cuticle and seal it shut. This not only assists with retaining moisture but it also gives the hair a healthy and shiny appearance.

pH Balance Made Simple:

pH stands for the "power of the hydrogen atom." It measures acidity and alkalinity of solutions ranging from a scale of 0-14. The low end of the scale is acidic, the high end is alkaline, and a pH of 7.0 is neutral or what is considered "balanced." According to Dr. Llaila Afrika of "African Holistic Health"

"Skin and hair do not have a pH...The pH of cosmetics will not change the pH of the hair or skin because the hair and skin contain keratin, fatty acids, and other substances that adjust the pH. As long as the pH is not unusually high or low there is no pH problem...There is no such thing as a "pH balanced" product because a product's pH will change while it is on the shelf in the store and change when applied to the hair and skin."

As mentioned above, when solutions are too acidic or too alkaline this can cause problems. This may cause the strands of the hair to feel parched, frayed, and have a dry appearance. However, while most products on the market may not be "ph balanced", their levels are generally not unusually high or low. When purchasing products the focus should be on the ingredients and understanding how one's unique texture is supposed to feel. If it feels inconsistent with its general state of health; it may be time

to check the quality one's products.
Macherey Nagel testing strips can assist with identifying the ph levels of solutions. They are available for purchase on our website at: ***http://ihairnatural.com/ihn/black-natural-hair-type-4c/***
These strips can test any type of solution, ranging from your drinking water to your saliva. If saliva is on the acidic side it can be balanced by increasing the intake of alkaline foods such as apples, watercress, and spinach (most fruits and vegetables). This will improve the quality of one's hair and their health in general.

Hair Types and Products

The Andre Walker Hair Chart:
When it comes to products and styles for natural hair; one size does not fit all. Determining the characteristics of one's hair type will help guide them to what styles and products are most suitable for their hair.

Identifying one's hair type can be made simple with the use of a natural hair chart. Hart charts are merely *guides* to assist one with their hair care management. They are not an exact science. Natural black hair is too diverse to be restricted to the limitations of a hair chart. However, hair charts are beneficial in that they can give one realistic expectations about their hair's capabilities. While there are several hair typing systems on the market, "The Andre Walker Hair Chart" is the most comprehensive. Andre Walker is the famous hairstylist to Oprah Winfrey. He was the first to develop a hair typing system and most other charts are modeled after his system.

This hair chart consists of four common hair types with a focus on its curl pattern. It ranges from "Type 1" to "Type 4" with corresponding subcategories of a, b, and c. This chart is excellent for giving one a general idea about how certain styles and products will turn out on their hair. Given the diversity of natural black hair, an individual may be a combination of two different hair types.

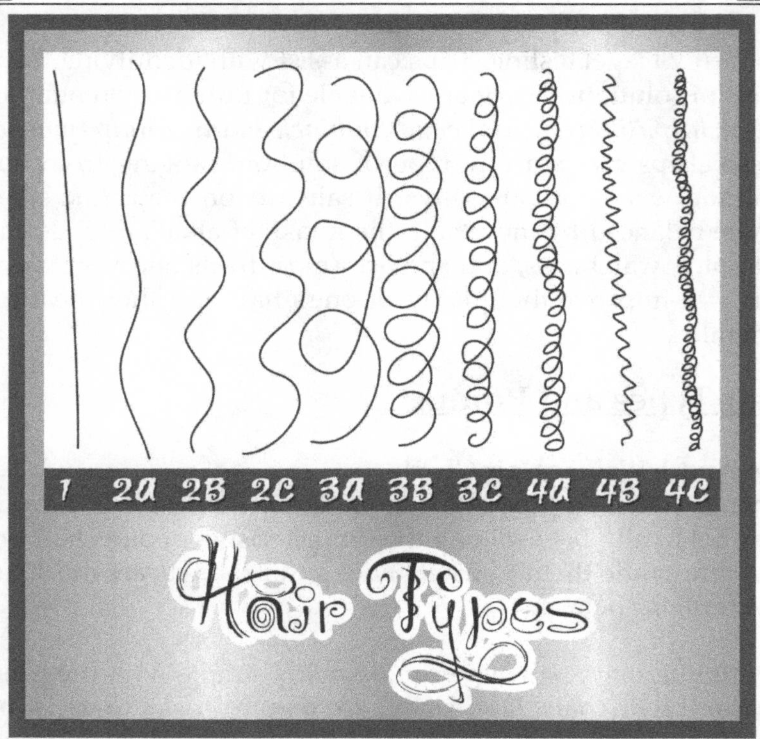

How to Identify Your Hair Type:

How one determines their hair type can begin by first washing their hair and rinsing it with cold water. Next, section off parts of the hair and look for the most common curl pattern. From this point, one can determine the shape of their curl pattern and match it to a particular hair type on the hair chart.

Once a hair type has been identified one can research what types of styles or products work best for their hair. A general rule of thumb when it comes to products is the tighter the curl pattern, the more moisture it requires. Further, lightweight products are more suitable for hair that is thin in density, and medium to heavier products are best suited for hair that is medium or thick in density. This will ensure that thin hair is not weighed down, and that thick hair is properly hydrated and moisturized.

Natural Hair Type 1: Straight Hair

Technically there is no such thing as natural hair type 1. While there are some aboriginal women that may have hair that closely resembles straight hair, the only way for Black women to achieve bone straight hair is through the use of chemical relaxers. Even if someone has a relaxer, and therefore an appearance of straight hair, they should still manage their hair according to their natural texture. Using products that cater to one's natural hair will ensure that they do not rob their hair of its much needed moisture which commercial products for straight hair have a tendency to do.

As new growth comes in one can do a strand test to see where their hair falls on the natural hair chart. They can conduct their hair care regimen based on that hair type. However, since the hair is technically straight and not as dense as tightly packed curly or kinky hair, it would work well with the use of lightweight moisturizers and oils like almond oil, coconut oil and safflower oil. **These products, along with a full listing of products for Natural Hair Type 1 can be purchased on our website at:** ***http://ihairnatural.com/ihn/black-natural-hair-type-1/***

Natural Hair Type 2A: Wavy Hair

Natural Hair Type 2A is hair that has a slight wavy curl pattern, and is medium to thin when it comes to density. This hair type is relatively easy to manage in comparison to other hair types along this hair chart. It is not too far removed from straight hair and therefore it is not prone to tangling or drying like tightly coiled natural hair. This hair type can be easily worn straight with the use of a blow dryer or flat iron. It can also be worn in its natural wavy state. However, due to its slip factor, it may not be able to hold certain styles like those along the nature of Type 3 and Type 4 hair.

Given the nature of this curl pattern it can be weighed down with heavy products, therefore lightweight to medium moisturizers and conditioners are most optimal. This hair type is best managed with frequent washing or at least once a week in order to prevent product build up. It is also best as with any hair type to use natural products, including shampoos free of harsh cleans-

ing agents like sulfates which will strip the hair of its natural oils. While this hair type does not have difficulty maintaining moisture it is still best to use products that provide moisture in order to maintain an adequate moisture balance.
Products like safflower oil, and "Cha' Cha All Natural Ultra Conditioning Sulfate-Free Shampoo" for dry, curly, wavy, kinky, and chemically treated hair is excellent for this hair type. **For a full listing of products for Natural Hair Type 2A please visit our website at: *http://ihairnatural.com/ihn/natural-hair-type-2a/***

Natural Hair Type 2B:
Natural Hair Type 2b is another subcategory of Type 2 hair. It is still wavy like Type 2a hair however, it forms more of a distinctive curl pattern where the "S" formation is easily identifiable. This hair type can vary in texture but in general it appears to range from either being thin to medium in density. It also has a tendency to get frizzy in humid weather.

As similar to Type 2A hair, Natural Hair Type 2b is more suited for light weight products and moisturizers. Natural oils like sunflower or sesame oil are excellent options because they are lightweight, high in vitamins A and E, and are excellent emollients which help to retain moisture in the skin and hair. Further, sesame oil has been used in traditional medicine to help alleviate stress, therefore it not only nourished the hair but aids in improving one's overall wellness.
These products can be purchased on our website along with a list of products that are suitable for this hair type at: *http://ihairnatural.com/ihn/natural-hair-type-2b/*

Natural Hair Type 2C:
Natural Hair Type 2c has deeper and thicker waves, than Type 2b hair. It also closely resembles Type 3 hair. This hair type falls between being both wavy and curly, therefore in terms of styling, someone with natural hair Type 2c hair can refer to styles on Type 2 and Type 3 hair. However, given that it has a tighter curl pattern than the other hair types that precede it on the chart, it is more prone to dryness, and tangles. It requires adequate moisture in order to prevent tangling and moisture loss.

Products that are suitable for both thin and medium textured hair are excellent choices for this hair type. Products such as "Kinky Curly Come Clean Natural Moisturizing Sulfate-free Shampoo", and "Hugo Naturals Balancing Conditioner" with tea tree and lavender oils work wonderfully for this hair type. **These products can be purchased on our website along with a list of products that are suitable for Natural Hair Type 2C at:** ***http://ihairnatural.com/ihn/natural-hair-type-2c/***

Natural Hair Type 3A: Curly Hair

Natural Hair Type 3A is where the strands of hair shift from wavy to curly. Type 3 hair in general falls right in the middle of the hair chart because it has the springy curl pattern of Type 4 hair, but it also has a texture that falls more closely to Type 2 hair. This hair type has a looser curl pattern within the type 3 spectrum which can be worn curly or straight with less heat or resistance than type 4 hair. However, it requires ample moisture just like Type 4 hair because it is much more difficult for sebum to penetrate the entire shaft of curly hair. Moisture has to be added to curly hair to keep it soft and manageable.

Given that curly hair has a tendency to become dry; co-washing with a moisturizing conditioner can be of great value. This limits the hair's exposure to sulfates which are commonly found in commercial shampoos.

Medium textured products like oils, creams or butters will work wonderfully with this hair type. When selecting products choose ones that also contain protein, as this will help to maintain the proper moisture/protein balance. If oils are a product of choice, natural oils that are derived from seeds or nuts like almond oil, or brazil nut oil will provide the hair with adequate protein and assist with sealing moisture into the hair.
These products can be purchased on our website along with a list of products that are suitable for Natural Hair Type 3A at: ***http://ihairnatural.com/ihn/black-natural-hair-type-3a/***

Natural Hair Type 3B:

Natural Hair Type 3b has a very defined curl pattern with a slightly looser curl than Type 3c hair. This hair type can vary dramatically in terms of texture and density, but the common factor is that curly hair, no matter what type or texture requires a lot of moisture. It is best to use moisturizers or conditioners that contain humectants, like honey, glycerin or aloe vera gel. Avoid the toxic or unnatural humectants like propylene glycol, which is an ingredient that is also used in brake fluid and anti-freeze

Sample Natural Hair Recipe
Medium weight moisturizers or natural oils are suitable for this hair type, or a blend of both is optimal. This recipe serves as an excellent product to seal moisture into the hair. The ingredients can be lightly warmed so that the shea butter can melt and blend into the mixture. Rewarm the product for reuse as needed. Further, when it solidifies it can also double as a nourishing lip balm.

- ¼ cup of olive oil
- ¼ cup of jojoba oil
- ⅛ cup of shea butter

These products can be purchased on our website along with a list of products that are suitable for Natural Hair Type 3B at:
http://ihairnatural.com/ihn/natural-hair-type-3b/
http://ihairnatural.com/ihn/hair-care-regimens/hair-oil-for-natural-black-hair/

Natural Hair Type 3C:
Natural Hair Type 3c is hair that is very curly. Its curl pattern is much more distinctive than the other Type 3 subcategories. This is where the natural curl starts to shift into looking like little springs or coils. It is also very similar in nature to Type 4a hair however, it my not be as course in texture.

This hair type requires ample moisture, and low manipulation is ideal when it comes to styling. This will help to keep the hair properly hydrated and prevent breakage as well. This hair type has a myriad of options when it comes to styling. It can be worn curly, braided, or straight. However it is not advised to straighten this hair often to lessen damage to the cuticle of the hair.

A pre-poo or co-washing method with a sulfate-free product

will help this hair type to retain its moisture. When it comes to conditioning and moisturizing this hair type works well with medium to heavy products like olive oil soap, cocoa butter, and cold pressed castor oil.
These products can be purchased on our website along with a list of products that are suitable for Natural Hair Type 3C at: ***http://ihairnatural.com/ihn/black-natural-hair-type-3c/***

Natural Hair Type 4A: Kinky Hair
According to the Andre Walker hair chart, Natural Hair Type 4A is where the hair begins to shift from being curly to "kinky." Kinky hair has an exceptionally defined curl pattern. Natural Hair Type 4a has curls that give an appearance of little tiny springs or coils stemming from the scalp of the hair. This hair type has an array of textures ranging from cottony, spongy, to wiry or course. Its density ranges from thin to thick.

Due to the nature of these curls, moisture is especially important to this hair type, and Type 4 hair in general. Washing can be done regularly with a sulfate free shampoo, however co-washing is highly recommended. This hair type can also benefit greatly from deep conditioning treatments to help deliver moisture to the cortex of the hair. This will help to make the hair more soft and supple, and prevent drying and breakage. Further, sleeping with a silk bonnet or pillowcase will aid in preventing moisture loss and breakage as well.

Natural hair type 4a is not limited when it comes to styling. It can be worn in curly and straight styles. However, low manipulation and protective styling will help to retain its length. Products like Carol's Daughter's "Healthy Hair Butter", and "Monoi Repairing Sulfate-Free Shampoo" work well with this hair type. **These products can be purchased on our website along with a list of products that are suitable for Natural Hair Type 4A at:** ***http://ihairnatural.com/ihn/natural-hair-type-4a/***

Natural Hair Type 4B:
Natural Hair Type 4b has curls that are a shade tighter than Natural Hair Type 4a. Its curls can also have a "Z" formation or an accordion appearance. The density of this hair type can range

from thick to thin, but it is not as fine or slippery as textures in Hair Types 1-3. While this hair type must be handled with care it is actually very strong. Having the ability to naturally coil and have a snap-back like quality shows just how resilient that naturally tightly coiled hair is.

When worn in its natural state, this hair type is not as adversely affected by wind or rain like other hair types that may frizz or lose their style when exposed to certain elements. Combating dryness is its biggest challenge, therefore moisture retention is key. Co-washing with a quality conditioner is recommended, and products that are heavier and more oil based are excellent to use to seal in moisture.

While this hair still requires adequate protein, a little goes a long way. Too much protein will cause this hair type to have a crunchy and dry texture. Heat should be applied at a minimum in order to maintain the health of this hair type. Products such as Curl Junkie's "Hibiscus & Banana Deep Fix Moisturizing Conditioner", and Curls' "Lavish Curls Moisturizer" are excellent products for this hair type. **These products can be purchased on our website along with a list of products that are suitable for Natural Hair Type 4B at: *http://ihairnatural.com/ihn/natural-hair-type-4b/***

Natural Hair Type 4C:
Natural Hair Type 4c is the last on the list of the Andre Walker Hair Chart. This hair type has a very tight curl pattern. This curl pattern as well as most curly hair, closely resembles the number 9 formation of "9 Ether Hair." Its texture and density can be diverse ranging from thin and spongy to thick and course.

This hair type requires a generous amount of moisture, therefore applying a moisturizer daily may benefit this hair type greatly. Type 4c hair is very strong but it must be handled with care. It is best to avoid using unnatural ingredients or combing this hair type unless it is wet.

Pre-poos and co-washing are highly recommended as cleansing methods to help retain moisture in the hair. This should be followed by an adequate intake of water to keep the entire system hydrated. Type 4c hair has difficulty holding shine due to its extremely tight curl pattern, therefore the pH levels of one's products should be checked to ensure that they are not unusually high or low. Some products like black soap fall on the high end of the alkaline scale (pH of 10.0). This raises the cuticle of the hair and causes it to lose moisture. It also gives the hair a dry and frayed appearance. While black soap is a wonderful natural product, its best if used occasionally on the hair as a clarifying shampoo followed by a moisturizing conditioner.

Medium to heavy oils, creams or butters work well with this hair type. Products such as "Jamaican Black Castor Oil", and She Moisture's "Organic Coconut & Hibiscus Curl & Shine Shampoo" are great products for this hair type. **These products can be purchased on our website along with a list of products that are suitable for Natural Hair Type 4C at: *http://ihairnatural.com/ihn/black-natural-hair-type-4c/***

CHAPTER 9: STYLE GALLERY

On seven beams of light travels the Goddess Iris. She is the straddle of the rainbow delivering to us the intentions, will, sounds, and directives from the Gods of on high. She is the manifested glory of the divine expressing herself through the style, etiquette, grace, and funk of this world's most prized resource…women. Iris come down and make your art."

-Interpretation of the Goddess Iris by H. Yuya T. Assaan-ANU

This book has covered in detail the fundamental principals of how to maintain healthy natural hair, and the wellness of ones' entire being. Now one is equipped to explore certain styles that will give their curls their own unique form of expression. The following is a small sample of the iHairNatural.com community. Here one can find inspiration and styles for all hair types and textures as these stylists and naturals share their creativity, philosophy, and personal gems as it pertains to the beauty of black natural hair.

At the iHairNatural.com community gallery one can find inspiration and styles for all hair types and textures as these stylists and naturals share their creativity, philosophy, and personal gems as it concerns the beauty of black natural hair.

Visit "**ihairnatural.com/ihn/ hairstyles-gallery/**" and explore the ihairnatural.com gallery and find out how you can become a member of the ihairnatural.com community.

Promote your business, style, and love for natural hair as a member of our growing community

New Jersey Salons

Salon: Meko New York, Natural Hair Care Spa & Boutique
Location: South Orange, New Jersey
Owner: Simeko Watkins Hartley
Contact Information: http://www.mekonewyork.com

Salon Owner: Simeko Watkins-Hartley

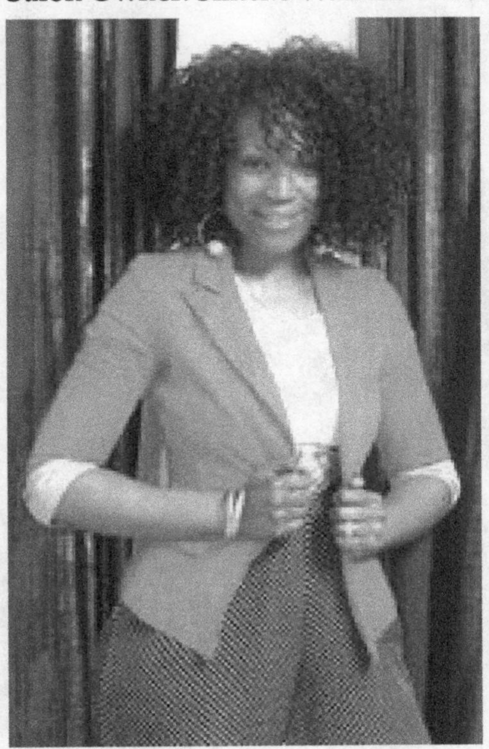

Meko New York's Philosophy:
"Our most important job as stylists is our commitment to educate our clients on how to properly care for their natural hair. Natural hair is like a delicate flower that needs to be watered (moisturized), nurtured and handled with care. Our natural hair is as unique as our finger print; no two heads of hair are the same. So we need to learn to embrace what we've been blessed with, have patience, and listen to your hair!"

All photos are courtesy of Simeko Watkins-Hartley

Style: Cornrows w/ Twist on the Side
Model: Chevonese Dublin

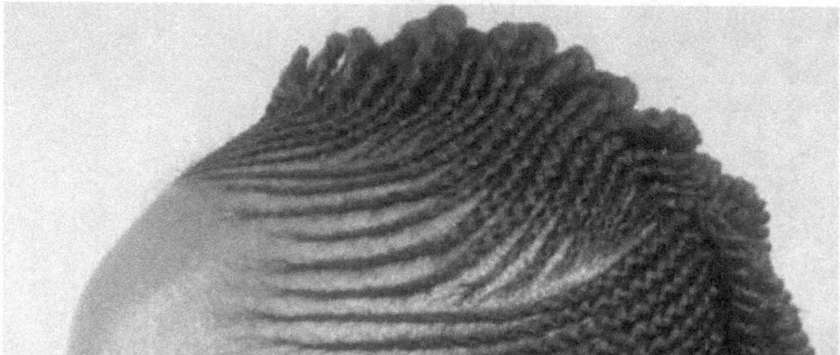

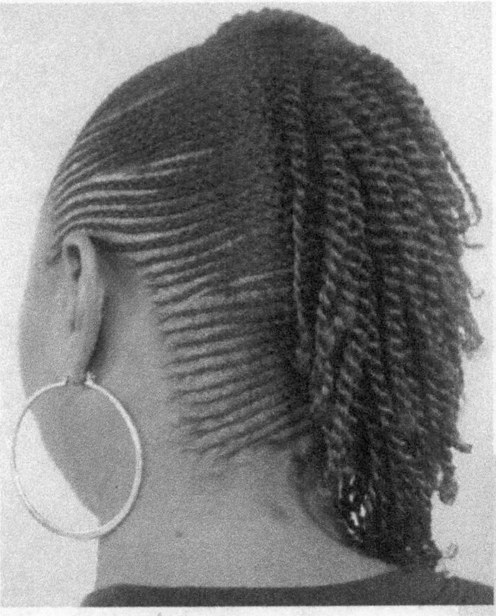

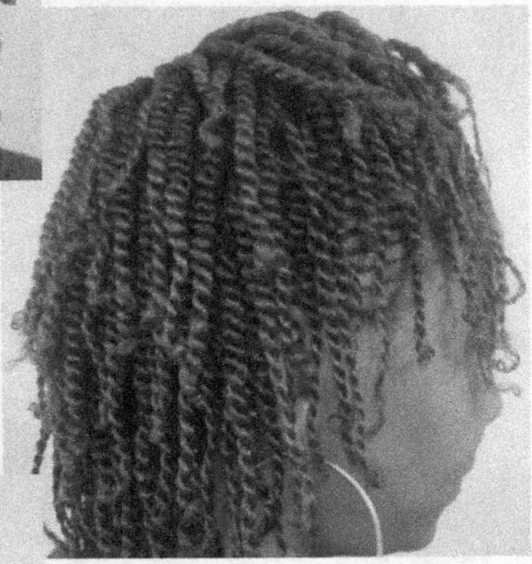

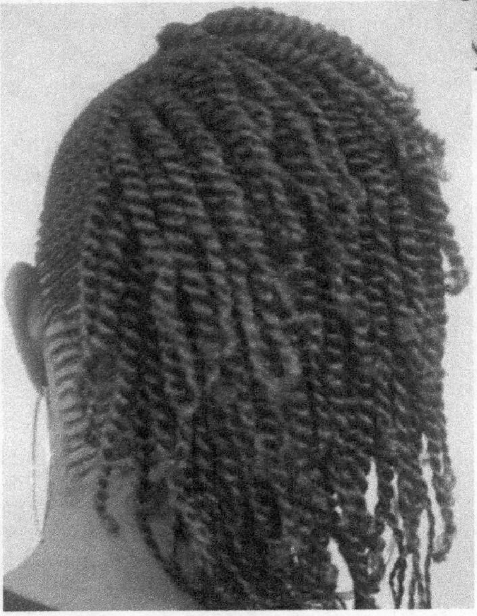

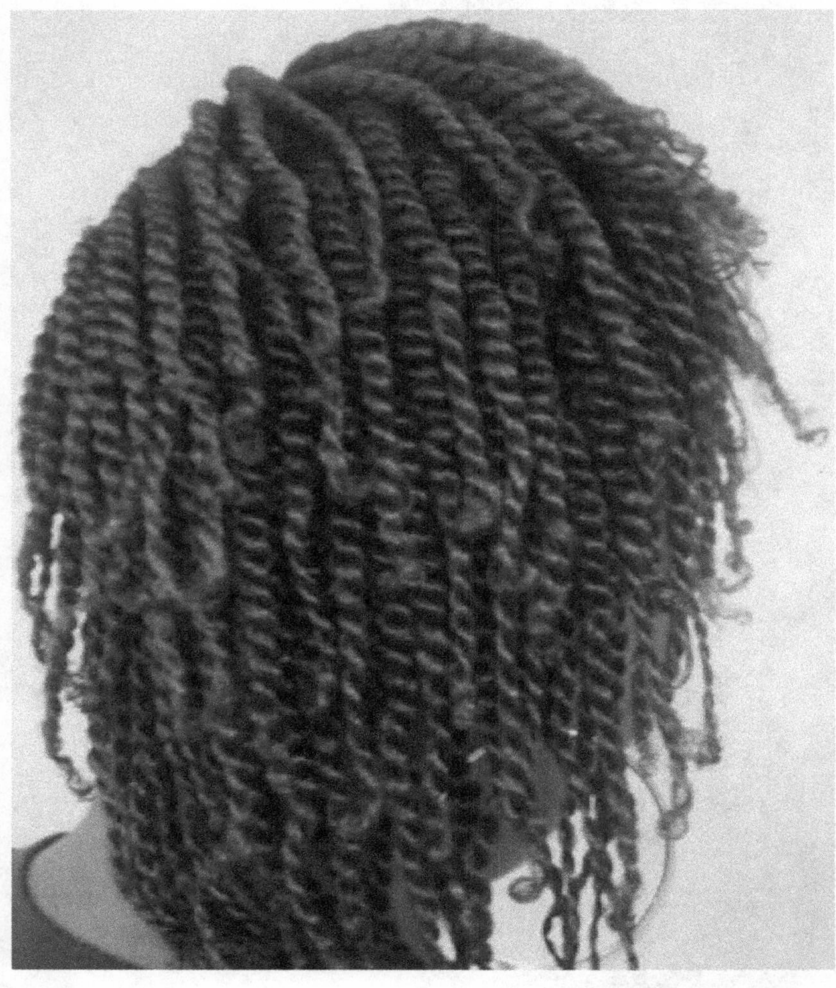

Style: Cornrow Up-do
Model: Aljamil Thomas

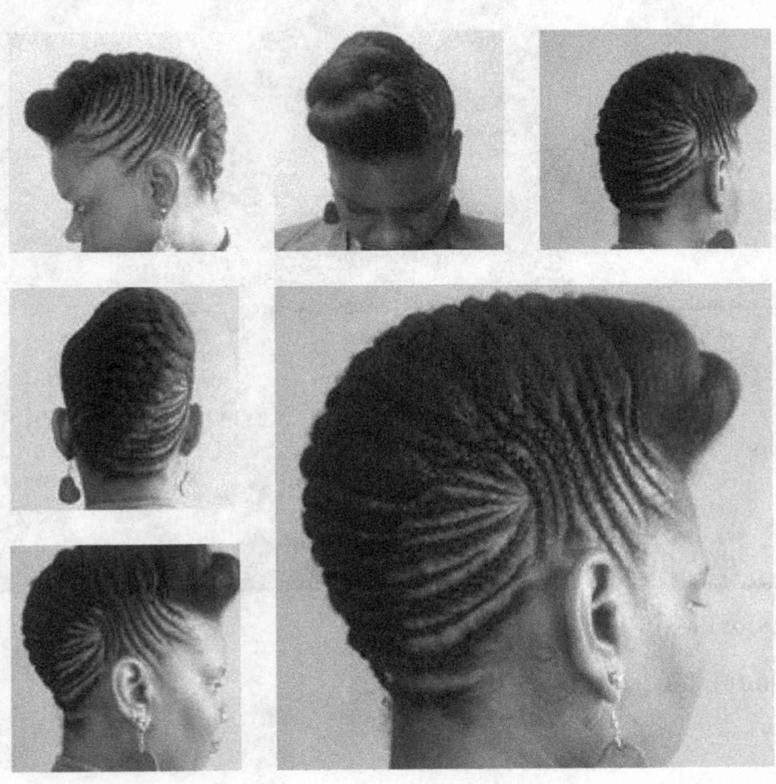

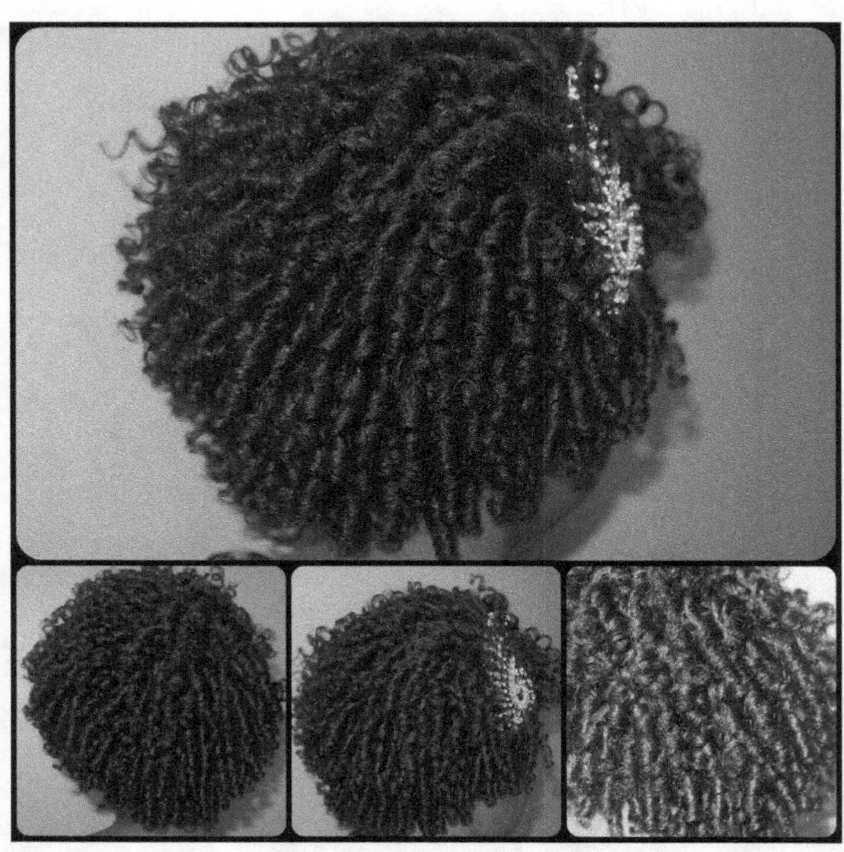

Style: Flexi Rod Set

Model: Jehanne Exe

SALON: STUDIO PURE

Location: Upper Montclair, New Jersey
Owner: Ahava Felicidad, The Holistic Hair Healer™
Contact Information: http://ahavafelicidad.wordpress.com/
Salon Owner: Ahava Felicidad, The Holistic Hair Healer™

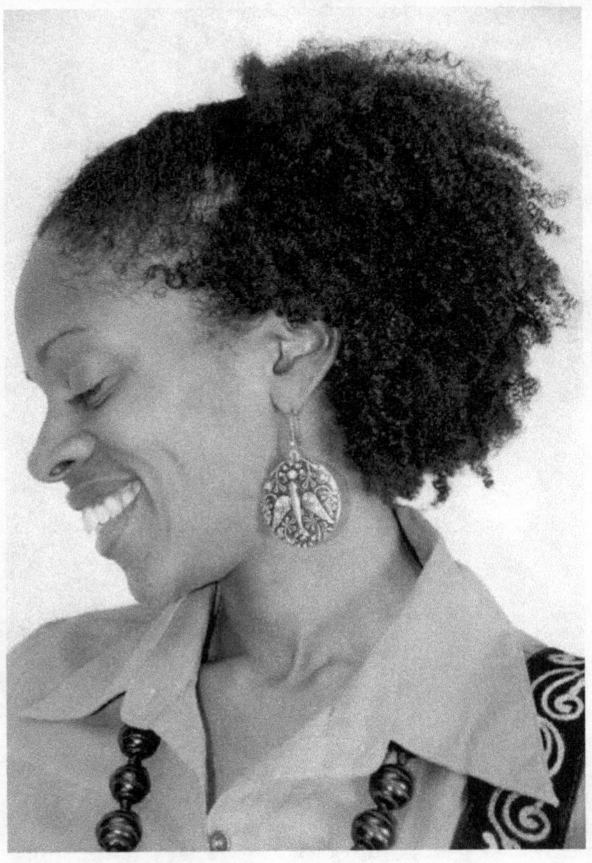

Studio Pure's Philosophy:
"Having natural hair is the freedom to be who you are – your whole self. Natural hair is versatile and unlimited as well as a healthy alternative to chemical processing."

All photos are courtesy of Ahava Felicidad

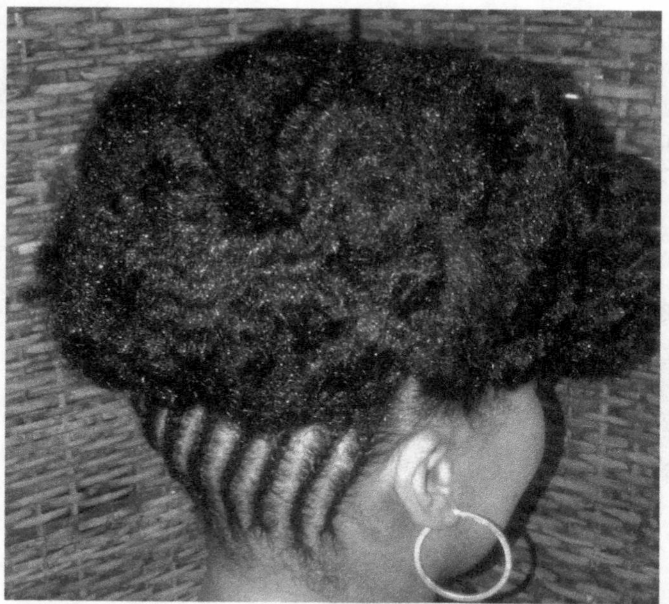

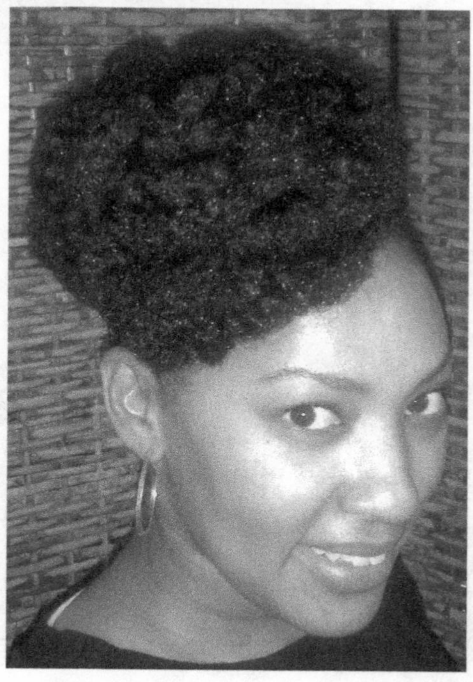

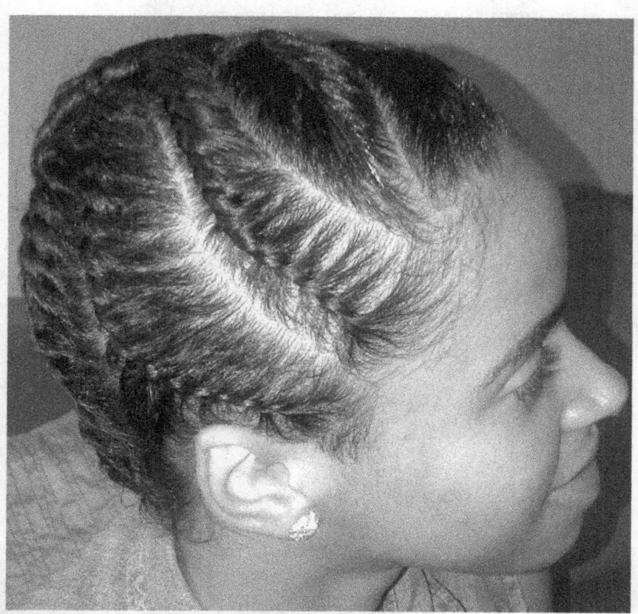

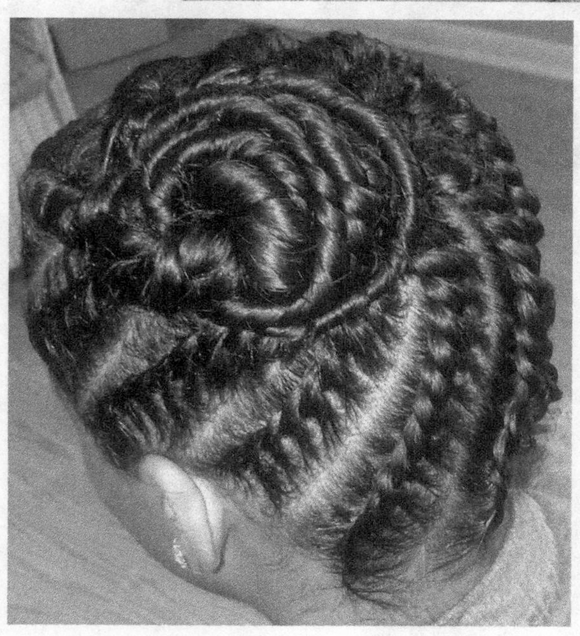

New York Salons

Salon: Locs of Nu Natural Hair Spa LLC,
Location: Brooklyn, New York
Owner: Ebony Nichols
Contact Information: http://locksofnunaturalhairspa.com/Home.html

Locs of Nu Natural Hair Spa LLC's Philosophy:
"We believe that we can and are, healing the community, follicle by follicle."

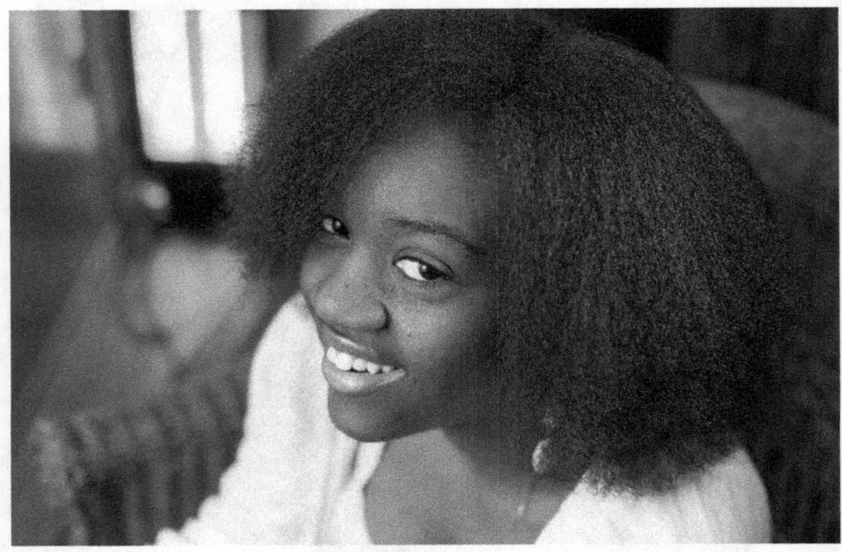

Photos courtesy of Raoul Gilles of Piknatural

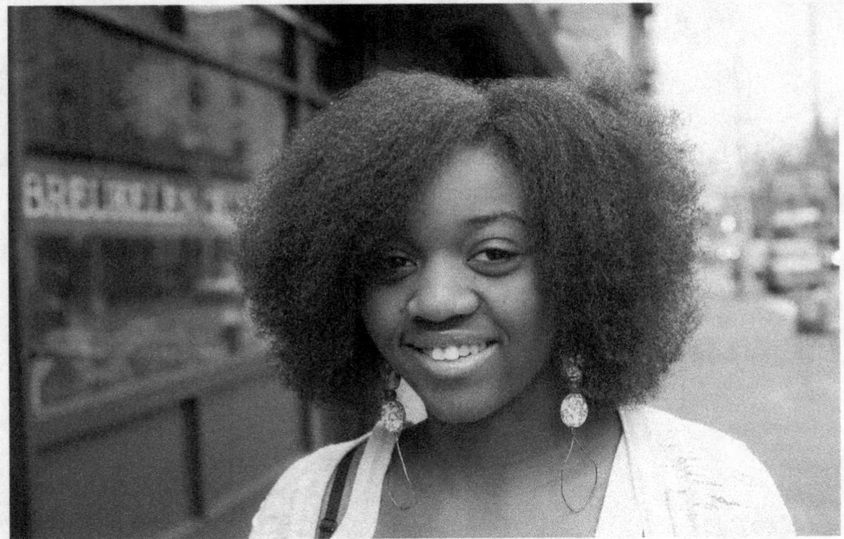

"I wear my hair natural because it shows who I am, and where I come from. It reminds people that Black, African Americans are unique as well." **Shavonna Hammond**

Arizona Salons

Salon: Hairloks by Arlette, Natural Hair Care Salon
Location: Scottsdale, Arizona
Owner: Arlette Pender
Contact Information: Hairloksbyarlette.com
Salon Owner: Arlette Pender

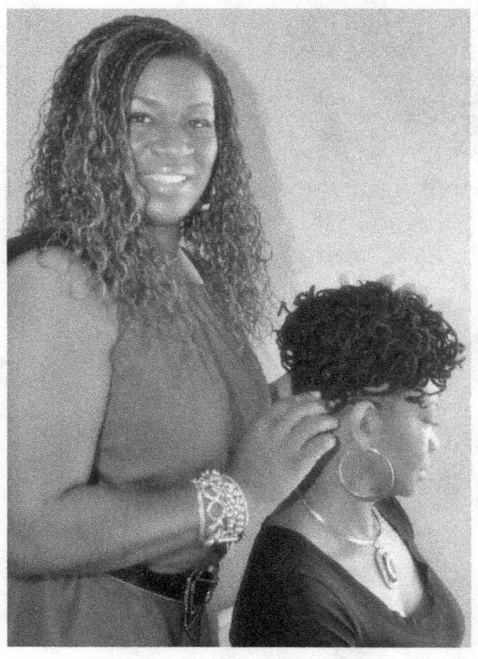

Hairloks Philosopy:
"Embrace your natural curl. Everyone's curl pattern is unique. Your hair is an outer expression of the inner you! Your hair is BEAUTIFUL!"

Photos Courtesy of Arlette Pender

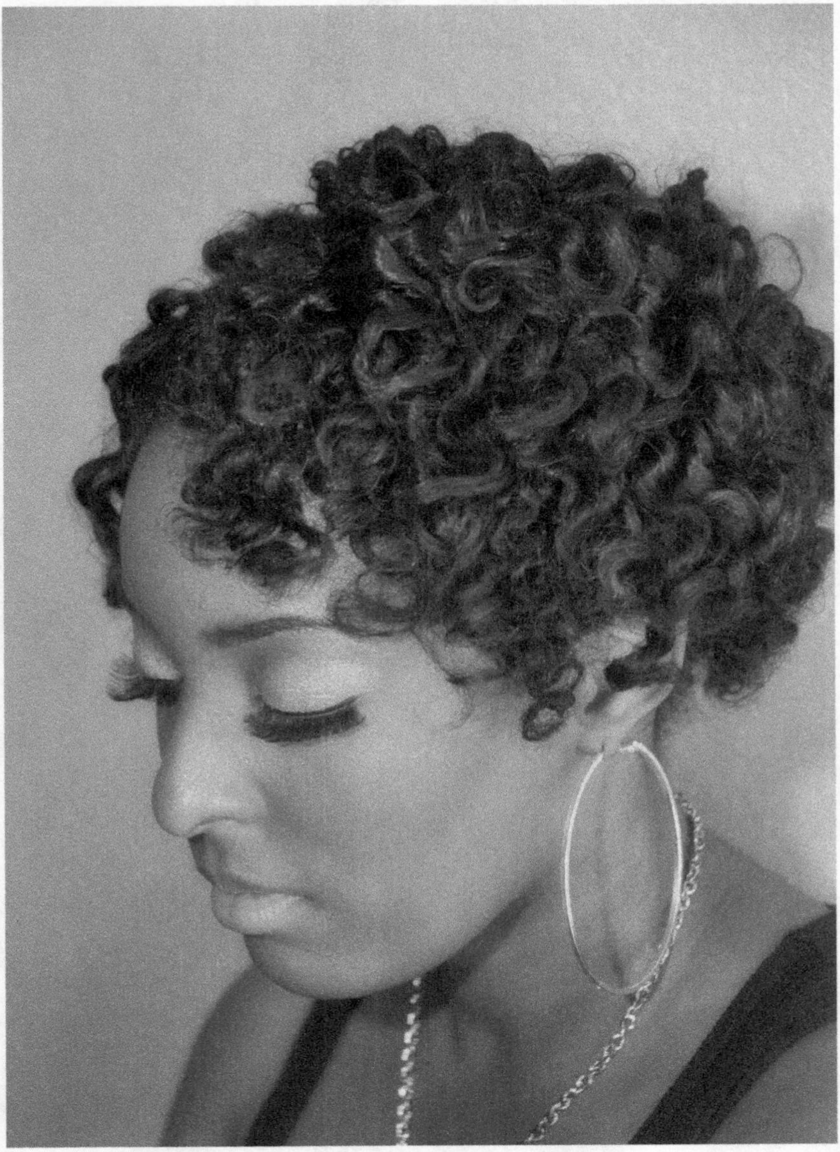

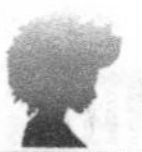

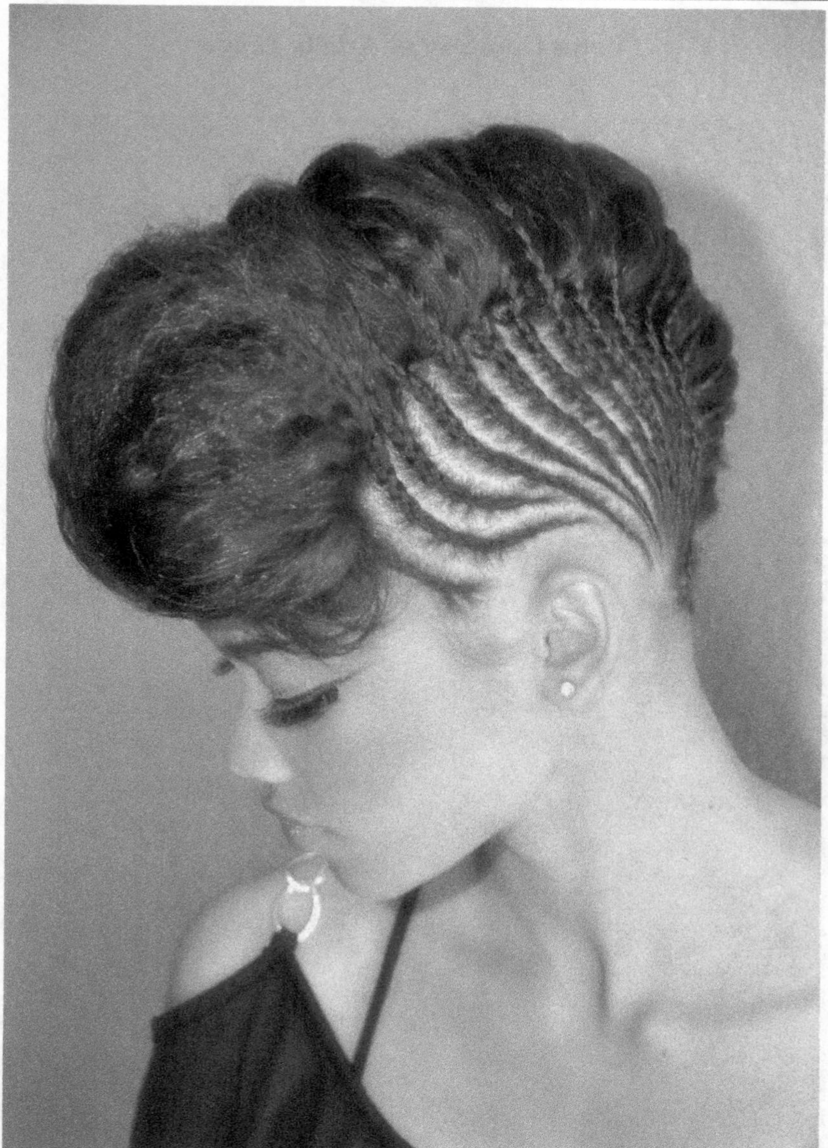

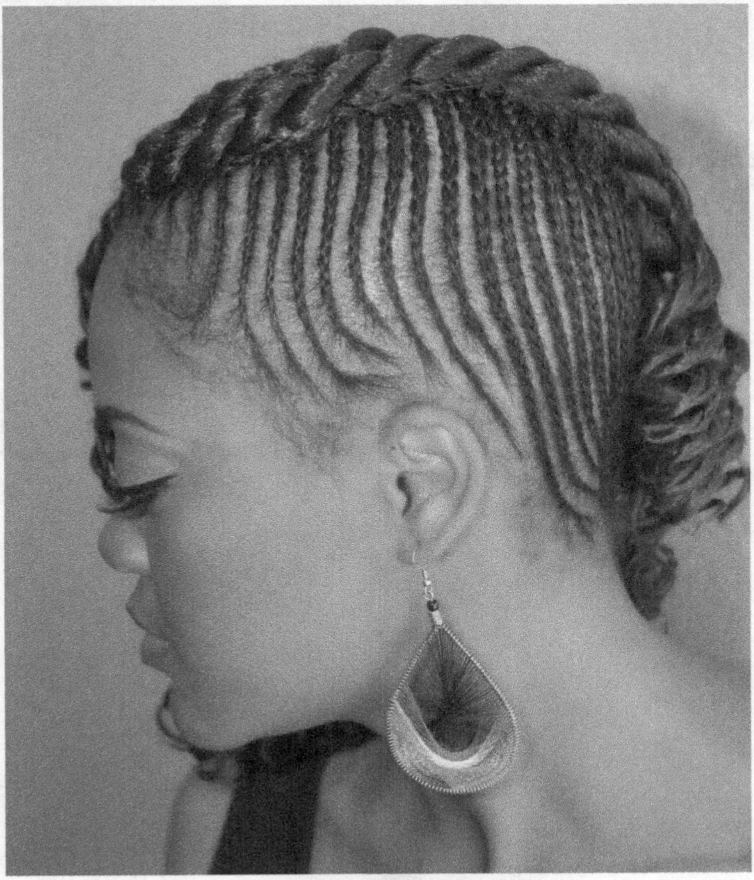

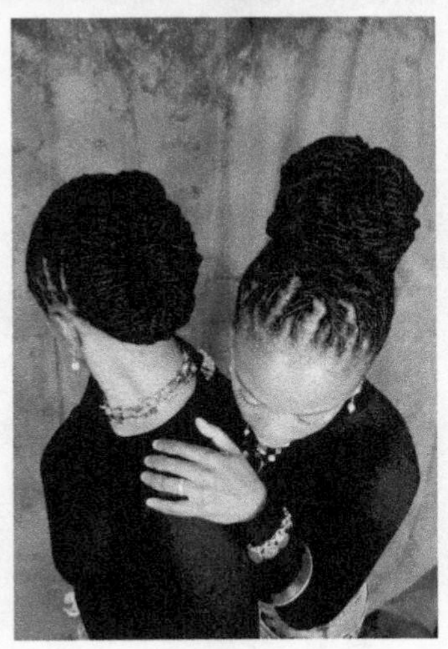

Tennessee Salons:

Salon: Kinky Rootz Salon

Location: Nashville, Tennessee

Owner: Kristi Alderson

Contact: Information : https://www.facebook.com/KinkyRootz

Kinky Rootz' Philosophy:

"Many people have misconstrued views on what it means to wear your hair natural. Natural is defined as "not affected, not artificial…like real life." Kinky Rootz Natural Hair Salon was created to revitalize individuals' with "chemical free tresses"

Photos Courtesy of Kristi Alderson

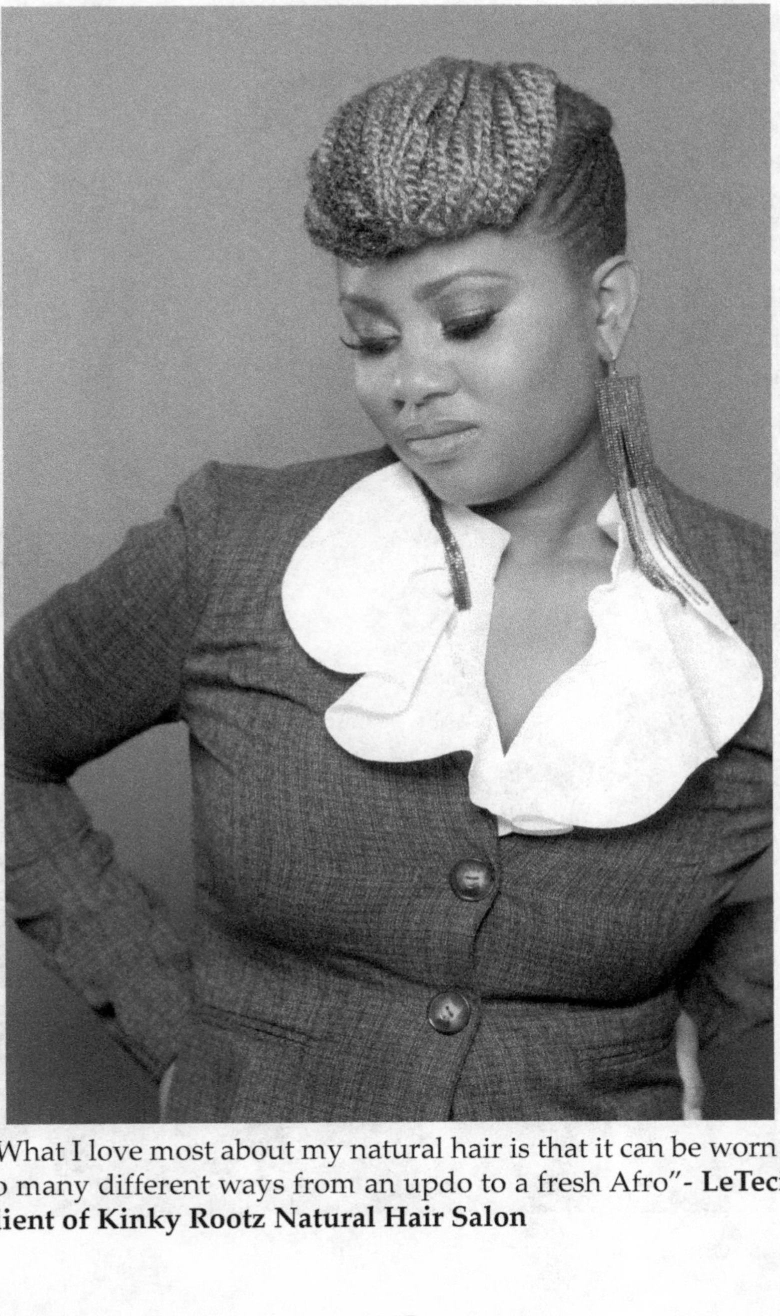

"What I love most about my natural hair is that it can be worn in so many different ways from an updo to a fresh Afro"- **LeTecia, client of Kinky Rootz Natural Hair Salon**

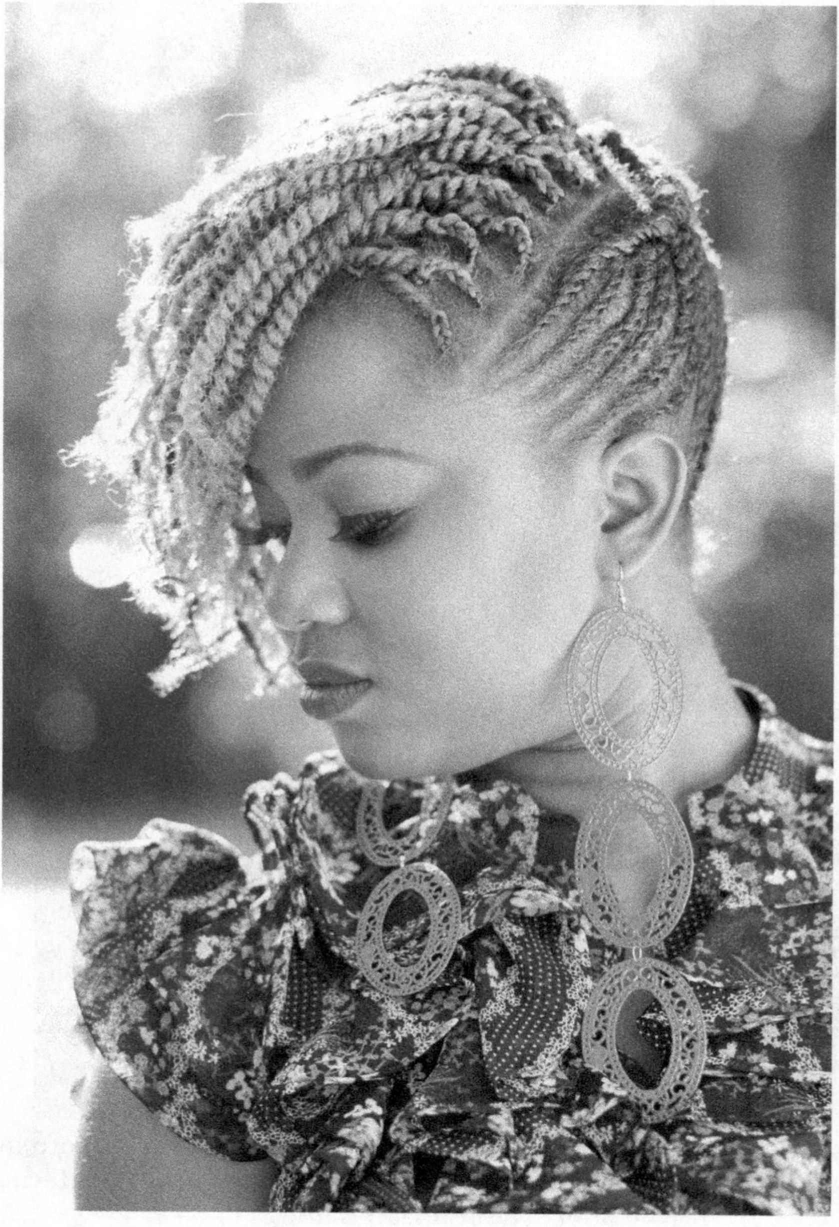

California Salons

Salon: Hairstory Natural Hair Salon
Location: Rancho Cucamonga, California
Owner: Imani Nash-Bey, Owner and Senior Certified Sisterlock Consultant
Contact Information: http://www.facebook.com/Hairstorynaturalhair

Hairstory's Philosophy:
"Our hairstory has deep rooted history...We make sure that you are getting all the attention that you need to help you be a better you."

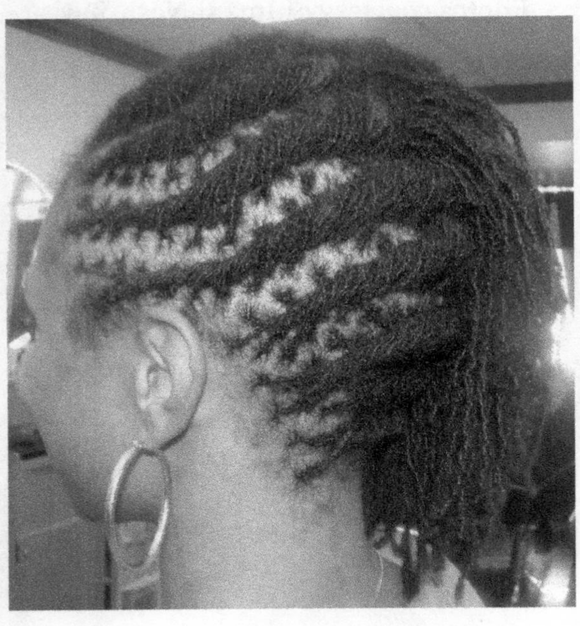

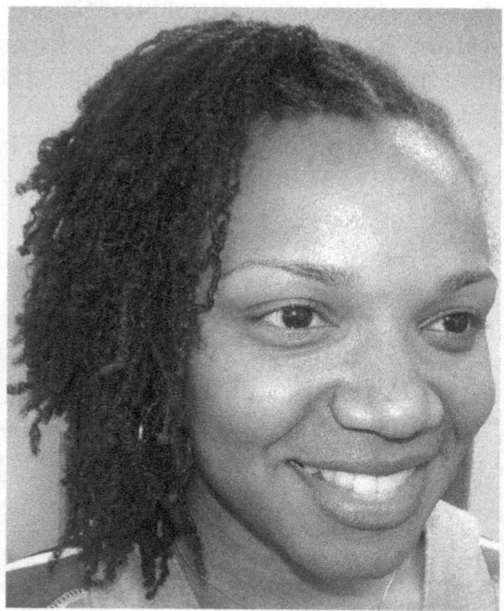

Photos courtesy of Imani Nash-Bey

Louisiana Salons

Salon: Beauty on de Bayou

Location: New Orleans, Louisiana
Owner: Dwana Makeba
Contact Information: http://www.beautyondebayou.com/

Photos Courtesy of Dwana Mekeba:

Dwana Mekeba: Salon Owner

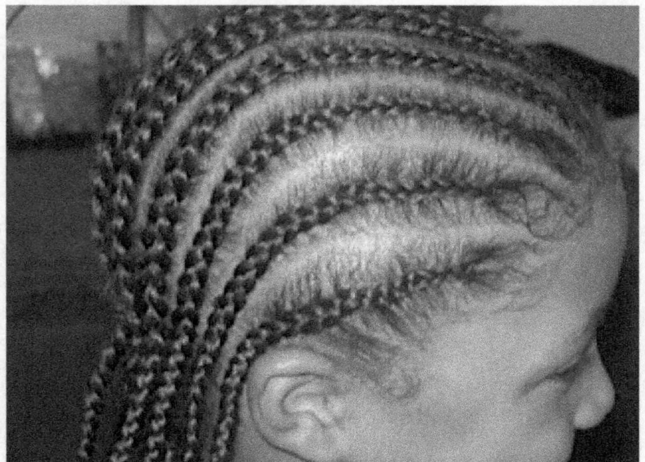

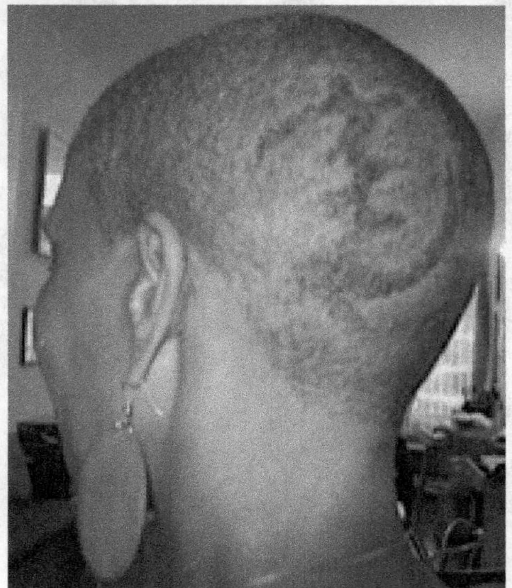

Beauty on de Bayou's Philosophy:
"Our mission is to provide a distinct atmosphere that offers the best quality service to our clients and to exhibit a positive image in the community. We provide chemical-free alternatives through the use of our hands as a tool, our eyes as a guide, and our heart and soul as inspiration."

Illinois Salons

Salon: Darya's Naturals
Location: Chicago, Illinois
Owner: Darya Johnson
Contact Information: http://www.daryanaturalhaircare.com/

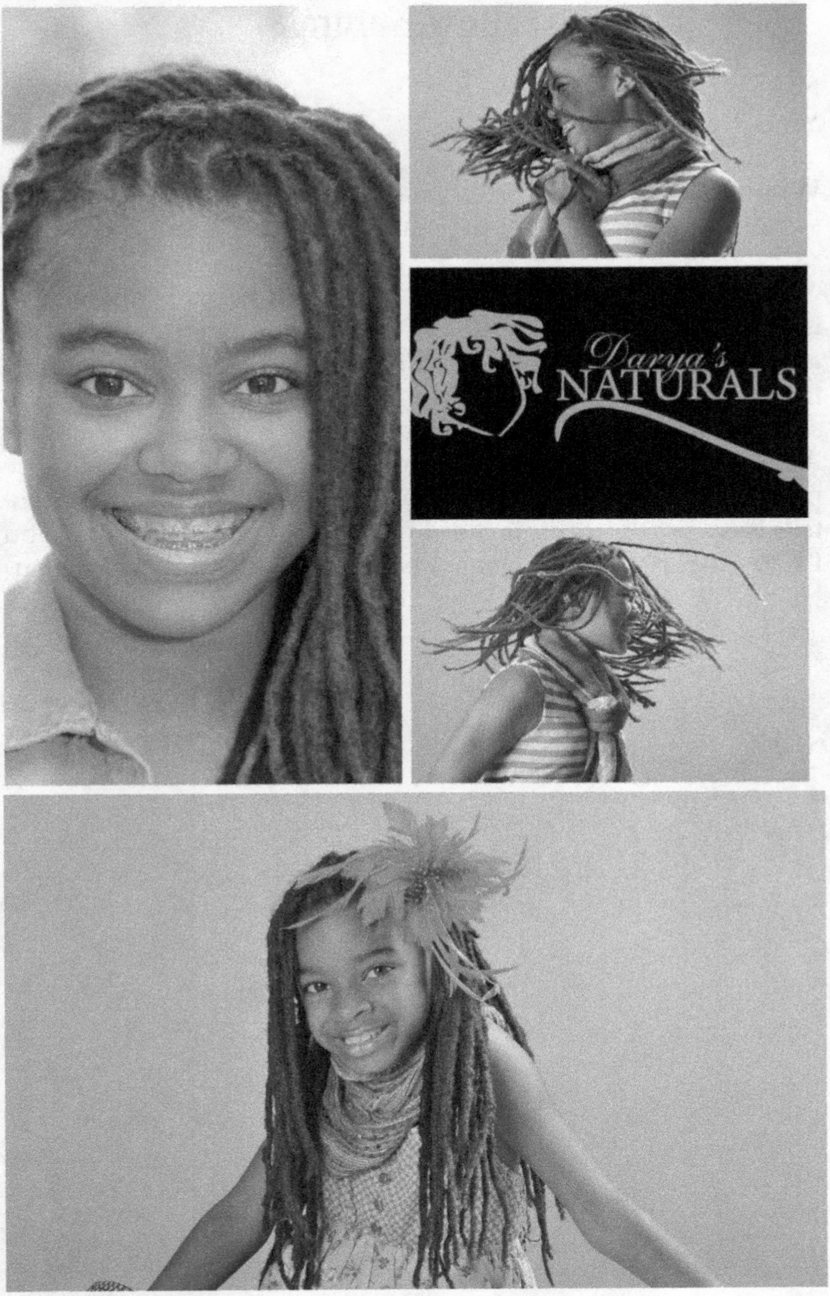

Darya's
NATURALS

Photos Courtesy of Darya Johnson

Fellow Naturals

Name: Tammy Wilson
Years Natural: 9 Years

What advice would you share to encourage our young women to see the beauty in embracing who they naturally are?
"While I prefer to encourage by example, I will tell anyone who is considering going natural that there are countless resources and support systems available. For most, being natural is not a fad. It is our reality. Because of this, many have had to build resistance against shade from friends, family, and even strangers. A person has to be mentally prepared for that...spiritually prepared to, unapologetically and with all due respect, show (and tell) the world that this is me. I would love for you to take it, but I'll be quite fine should you chose to leave it."- **Tammy Wilson**

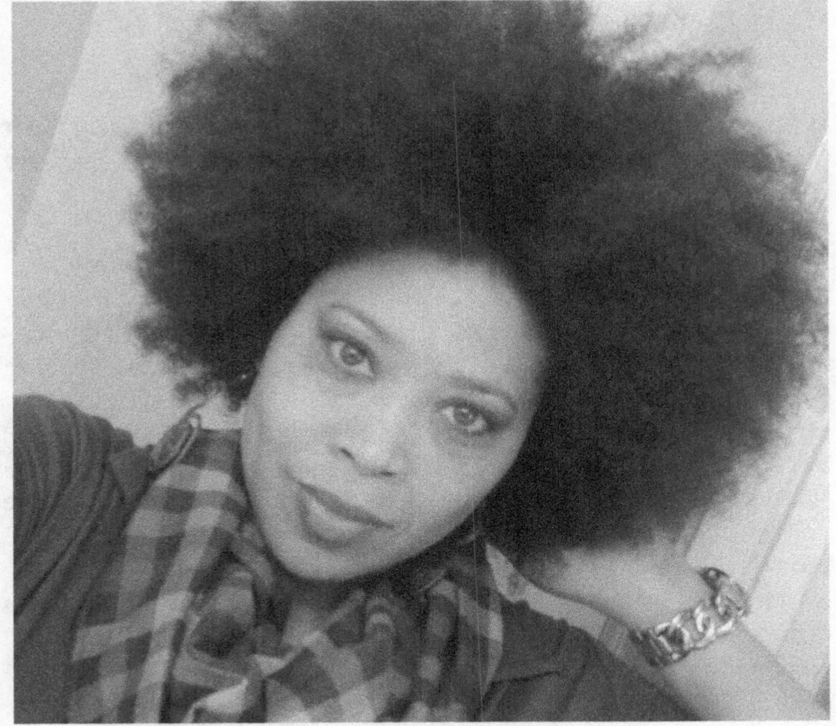

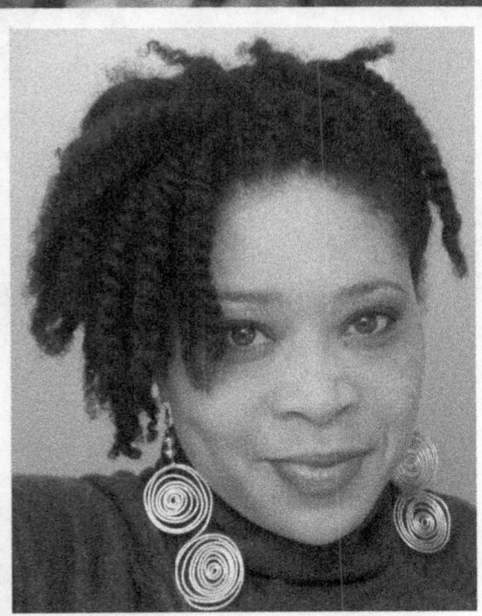

Photos courtesy of Tammy Wilson

Name: Ebony B. Cogdell
Years Natural: 6 ½ Years

What challenges did you encounter on your natural hair journey, and what solutions did you employ to remedy them?

"My most challenging moments involved some of my family and friend's initial reactions to my decision to become natural. Negative comments from parents, grandparents and even acquaintances affected me greatly. My advice for anyone experiencing verbal backlash would be to show them how fly natural hair can be. Yes, they may call you "Ceely" from The Color Purple, but show them how chic and stylish Ceely's natural hair can be. Many of the same people that questioned my decision to become natural now applaud me for it. Winning Taliah Waajid's 2012 World's Next Top Natural Hair Model contest was the ultimate comeback to my naysayers' disapproval. Not only did I get a chance to be a spokesperson for Black Earth products, but I also received a cash prize, free products, and the opportunity to connect and engage with prominent leaders in the Black hair care industry."
-Ebony B. Cogdell

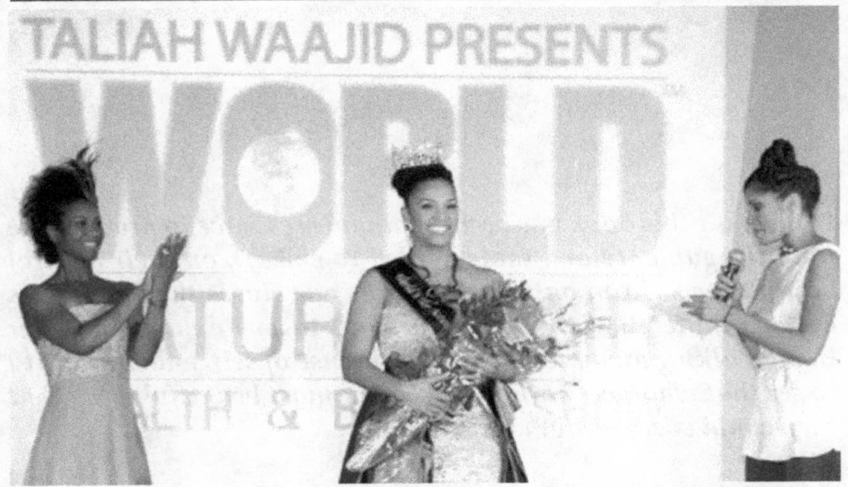

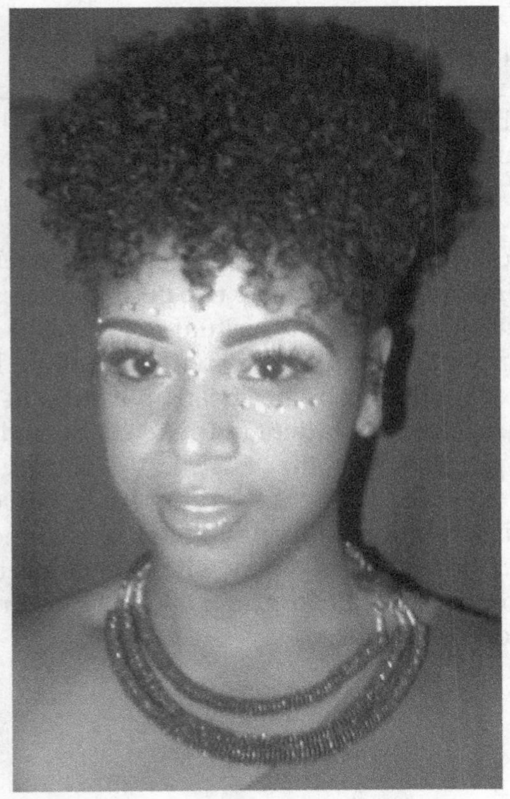

Photos Courtesy of Ebony B. Cogdel

I hope that this book has been a valuable resource to provide one with the guidance and tools needed to embark on their natural hair journey. I can only hope that as one closes the final pages of this chapter, that they open the pages to a new chapter of their lives; walking away with a renewed sense of self, and the ability to see that what one naturally is, is the most beautiful thing that they could ever possibly be.

About the author:
Phylecia is a natural hair blogger, author, and workshop teacher. As early as the age of 6 years old Phylecia learned how to braid and style hair, and later became the neighborhood stylist for friends and family members.

In 2011 when she decided to make the transition to return natural, that decision began to open her up to a new awareness which put her on a path to study African spiritual systems and metaphysics which she continues to study today with the Sadulu House Spiritual Institute. While she by no means purports herself to be a conscious guru, she is a student of the sciences, and has become aware of the programming that exists in this society that aims to keep our people sedated and dis-empowered. Phylecia's goal is to share this information with our young black women, so that at the very least, they will walk away with some tools to help them embrace who they naturally are, and take back control over their own mind, body and spirit.

FOR MORE INFORMATION ABOUT NATURAL HAIR CARE PLEASE COME VISIT US AT

WWW.IHAIRNATURAL.COM

If you are interested in being featured in an interview on our site, participating in our monthly focus groups, or participating in our upcoming natural hair show for young people, please come visit us at www.iHairNatural.com

Connect with Me Online:
iHairNatural.com
Twitter: twitter.com/iHairNatural
Facebook: Facebook.com/iHairNatural
Blogtalkradio.com/iHairNatural
ANU Publishing: Anu-BOOKSTORE.com

BIBLIOGRAGPHY

Afrika, Llaila O. African Holistic Health. Brooklyn, NY: A&B Publisher Group, 2004.

Afrika, Llaila. Nutricide. Brooklyn, NY: A&B Publisher Group, 2000.

Assaan-ANU, HRU Yuya T., ed. ANU Publishing, 2013

Assaan-ANU, HRU Yuya T. Grasping the Root of Divine Power: Anu Publishing, 2010

"Killed by Her Hair Extensions: "Woman Dies After Allergic Reaction 'To glue in Hairdo.'" Mail Online. 2 Feb. 2012. <http://www.dailymail.co.uk/health/article-2095450/Atasha-Graham-dies-allergic-reaction-glue-hairdo-night-out.html>

Kwatamani, High Priest. Raw and Living Foods. The KWATAMANI Holistic Institute of Brain Body & Spiritual research & Dev., Inc., 2008.

Littlefield, Amy. "Toxic Hair Treatment Highlights Need to Regulate Industry." Gender Across Borders. 26 Apr. 2011. <http://www.genderacrossborders.com/2011/04/26/toxic-hair-treatment-shows-need-to-regulate-beauty-industry/>

Melanin. Black Talk Radio 2011 <http://www.youtube.com/watch?v=qQ8XLqlvL6s>
Muhammad, Elijah. Message to the Blackman in America. Muhammad, Elijah, 1973

Pookrum, Jewel. Vitamins & Minerals from A to Z. Brooklyn, NY. A&B Publisher Group, 1999.

Reid, Daniel P. The Tao of Health Sex & Longevity. New York, NY. Fireside, 1989.

The Melanin Chronicals. 2011

Tse-Tung, Chairman Mao. The Quotations from Chairman Mao Tse-Tung the Little Red Book. Peking, Beijing. Foreign Languages Press, 1972.

Tudor-ANU, Aime., ed. ANU Publishing, 2013

Wise, Lauren A. et.al. "Hair Relaxer Use and Risk of Uterine Leiomyomata in African-American Women." American Journal of Epidemiology, Boston, MA. 12 Feb. 2012 http://aje.oxfordjournals.org/content/175/5/432

CPSIA information can be obtained
at www.ICGtesting.com
Printed in the USA
BVHW032044170521
607566BV00005B/129

9 780615 825885